Falls Handbook: Clinical and Medical-Legal Perspectives of Falls Across the Lifespan

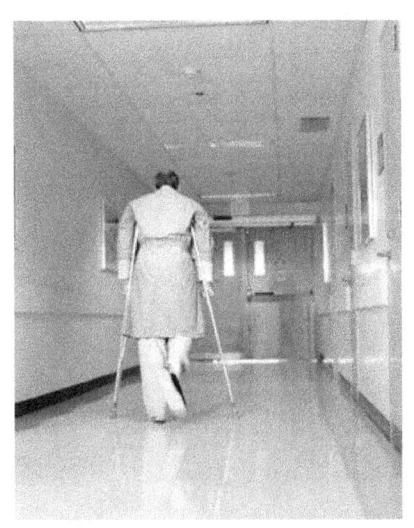

**Deanna Gray-Miceli, DNSc, APRN, FAANP,
Elizabeth Capezuti, PhD, RN, FAAN,
William T. Lawson, III, JD,
Patricia Iyer MSN, RN, LNCC**

www.legalnursebbusiness.com
11205 Sparkleberry Drive Fort Myers, FL 33913
Copyright 2007

Legal Nurse Consultants
www.legalnursebusiness.com

Falls Handbook: Clinical and Medical-Legal Perspectives of Falls Across the Life Span

Deanna Gray-Miceli
Elizabeth Capezuti
William Lawson
Patricia Iyer

Publisher: Legalnursebusiness.com
11205 Sparkleberry Drive,
Fort Myers, FL 33913

Cover Art: 908-391-7933

Ryan Sanchez

First Edition

Copyright 2007 by Legalnursebusiness.com

All rights reserved. No part of this publication may be reproduced, stored in a retrieval system, or transmitted, in any form or by any means, electronic, mechanical, photocopying, recording, or otherwise, without prior written permission from the publisher.

Permission to photocopy or reproduce solely for internal or personal use is permitted in libraries or other users registered with the Copyright Clearance Center, provided that the base fee of $4.00 per chapter plus $.10 per page is paid directly to the Copyright Clearance Center, 222 Rosewood Drive, Danvers, MA 01923. This consent does not extend to other kinds of copying, such as copying for general distribution, for advertising or promotional purposes for creating new collected works, or for resale.

ISBN 13: 978-1480086128

ISBN 10: 1480086126

Dedication

For my husband and daughter for your continual support, love and patience as this book developed; to those suffering from unexplained or serious falls and those professionals ministering care; to fellow citizens and to an insightful public health mentor and colleague.

Deanna Gray Miceli

Table of Contents

About the Authors I

Introduction III

Chapter One - Overview of Falls in America by Deanna Gray-Miceli 1-1

    A. National Imperatives 1-1

    B. Defining Falls 1-2

        1. Clinical perspective of patient falling 1-3
        2. A case definition perspective 1-5
        3. The researcher's perspective 1-5
        4. The falling person's perspective 1-5

    C. Fall Epidemiology: Magnitude, Scope and Economic Impact 1-6

        1. Overview of data sources 1-6
        2. Fatal fall incidences (children and older adults) 1-6
        3. Non-fatal fall incidences and injuries (children and older adults) 1-7
        4. Fatal fall incidence in the workplace 1-8
        5. Economic impact of falls 1-8
        6. Overview of incidence of falls in medical care settings 1-9

            a. Falls in the nursing home 1-9
            b. Falls in children's hospitals 1-9
            c. Falls in acute-care hospitals 1-10

    D. Consequences of Falls 1-10

        1. Overview of common injuries 1-10
        2. Hip fracture 1-11
        3. Traumatic brain injury 1-11
        4. Psychological injury 1-12

    E. Patterns of Falls and Their Significance 1-12

Chapter Two - The Multifactorial Nature of Falls by Deanna Gray-Miceli .. 2-1

    A. Factors Associated with Falls 2-1

    B. Indoor and Outdoor Public Environmental Hazards and Falls 2-1

    C. Environmental Hazards in and Around the Home and Their Assessment ... 2-2

       1. Falls associated with steps, ladders, or stools 2-3
       2. Falls in the bathroom 2-3
       3. Other hazardous areas 2-3

   D. Environmental Falls in Healthcare Settings 2-4

   E. Equipment Safety 2-6

   F. Medications Related to Falls 2-6

   G. Age-Related Changes Associated with Falling 2-6

   H. Medical Causes of Falls 2-7

   I. Intrinsic Risk Factors Associated with Falls for an Older Adult 2-7

   J. Risk Factor Assessment in the Medical Care Setting 2-8

Chapter Three – Prevention of Falls in the Hospital by Deanna Gray-Miceli and Elizabeth Capezuti 3-1

   A. General Issues Influencing Patient Safety and Quality Care 3-1

   B. Levels of Prevention 3-1

   C. Framework for Reducing Patient Falls (Adverse Events): Root Cause Analysis 3-3

       1. Defining error 3-3
       2. Process and components of root cause analysis 3-4

   D. Measures to Prevent Patient Falls 3-4

       1. Communication 3-5
       2. Documentation 3-6
       3. Environmental and equipment safety 3-7
       4. Fall risk assessment 3-8

           a. General issues related to measures of fall risk 3-8

   E. Fall Risk Assessment Versus Post-Fall Assessment 3-10

       1. Post-fall assessment 3-10
       2. Post-fall treatment 3-12

   F. General Issues to Consider Regarding Patient Falling 3-12

       1. Autonomy 3-12
       2. Medical stability 3-13

   G. Hospital Policies and Procedures for Fall Reduction 3-13

H. Prevention of Falls in the Institutionalized Patient 3-15

    1. Prevention of falls in the hospitalized elderly 3-15
    2. Prevention of falls in hospitalized children 3-16

Chapter Four - Prevention of Falls in Nursing Home Residents by Elizabeth Capezuti 4-1

A. Federal Regulations 4-1

B. Fall Risk Assessment in the Nursing Home 4-1

    1. The process and use of fall risk assessment tools 4-1
    2. Risk factors 4-2

C. Addressing Side Effects of Medications 4-4

D. Providing Appropriate Observation 4-5

E. Promoting Safe Mobility 4-8

F. Promoting Safe Transferring 4-9

G. Promoting Comfortable, Individualized Seating 4-10

H. Preventing Falls from Bed 4-12

Chapter Five - Physical Restraints and Side Rails by Elizabeth Capezuti 5-1

A. Introduction 5-1

B. Definition 5-1

C. Restraint/Side-Rail Related Injuries, Including Death 5-3

D. Recent Research/Clinical Practice Regarding the Relationship to Falls/Injuries 5-5

E. Standards Related to Use of Physical Restraints 5-6

Chapter Six – Legal Aspects of Falls by Elizabeth Capezuti, William Lawson and Patricia Iyer 6-1

A. The Legal Process 6-1
    1. Damages/injuries 6-1
    2. Caller's relationship to patient 6-1
    3. Caller's perceptions of what was done wrong 6-1
    4. Admissions and apologies 6-2
    5. Location of the fall 6-2
    6. Date of the fall 6-2

  B. Standard of Care as a Dynamic Concept 6-3

  C. Professional Policies and Guidelines 6-4

  D. Common Allegations in Fall Cases 6-4

  E. Evolution of the Suit 6-5

  F. Defense Theories 6-6

    1. Factual denial 6-6
    2. Patient care or injury was the responsibility of others 6-7
    3. Recognized complications 6-7
    4. Standard of care was followed 6-7
    5. Nursing judgment 6-8
    6. Two schools of thought 6-8
    7. Lack of proximate cause 6-8
    8. Contributory negligence of plaintiff 6-8
    9. Failure of plaintiff's expert to list a deviation from nursing practice 6-10

  G. Punitive Damages 6-11

    1. Pattern of substandard care 6-11
    2. Motivation to provide substandard care 6-11
    3. Profits 6-12
    4. Defense of punitive damages claims 6-12

Appendix AP-1

 Appendix One AP-1
  Check for Safety: A Home Fall Prevention Checklist for Older Adults AP-1

 Appendix Two AP-4
  Case One: Inaccurate Description of Fall AP-4
  Case Two: Dropped by Aides AP-6
  Case Three: Fall Down Stairs AP-11
  Case Four: Fall in Bathroom AP-13

About the Authors

Deanna Gray-Miceli, DNSc, APRN, FAANP is a consultant to New York University-John Hartford Institute for Geriatric Nursing (NYU-JHIGN), invited consultant to a state department of health for statewide fall prevention initiatives and on the faculty of Rutgers University, School of Nursing. As a doctorally prepared gerontological nurse practitioner for over 2 decades, Deanna has devoted her clinical and research interests to evaluation and care of older adults who fall. In the mid-1990s she founded and directed the first academic nurse managed Fall Assessment and Prevention Program in the country housed at a school of medicine. In 2001, she completed a doctoral degree focusing her dissertation research on the "Lived Experience and Meaning of a Serious Fall to Older Adults". In 2002, Deanna was awarded a two-year Post-Doctoral Scholarship by The John A. Hartford Building Academic Geriatric Nursing Capacity Program, working with faculty mentors from the School of Nursing and School of Medicine at the University of Pennsylvania.

Dr. Gray-Miceli's program of research includes the development, validation and feasibility for RNs to use a post-fall assessment tool for older adults in nursing homes who fall. The tool is capable of detecting reasons for fall events by clinical staff. To further test its clinical use and feasibility by clinical staff to reduce falls, Deanna was awarded a pilot grant through the Division of Long-Term Care Awards at the University of Pennsylvania School of Medicine.

Dr. Gray-Miceli's work in fall prevention includes nursing, interdisciplinary, and consumer education, clinical research and development of programs and services for older adults who fall. In 2006, she was an invited reviewer to the State and Territorial Injury Prevention Directors Association (STIPDA), Injury Surveillance Workgroup on Falls [ISW4] Report: Consensus Recommendations for Surveillance of Falls and Fall-related Injuries, and contributed to ECRI's book "Fall Prevention Strategies in Health Care Settings". Deanna has published over 25 refereed journal articles, 10 book chapters and presented over 25 papers or posters at national and local scientific meetings most related to falls in older adults. As a consultant to NYU, Deanna is Project Director to the AACN/JHI sponsored grant "Preparing Nursing Students to Care for Older Adults: Enhancing Gerontology in Senior-level Undergraduate Courses: The G-NEC Experience." Deanna is a Fellow of the American Academy of Nurse Practitioners and the Gerontological Society of America.

Elizabeth Capezuti, PhD, RN, FAAN is a BS graduate of Lehman College (1980), and an MSN graduate of Hunter College - Bellevue School of Nursing (Geriatric Nurse Practitioner, 1984). In 1995, she received her Ph.D. in Nursing from the University of Pennsylvania and is currently an Associate Professor and Co-Director of the John A. Hartford Foundation Institute for Geriatric Nursing at New York University College of Nursing. Dr. Capezuti has published extensively in the areas of fall prevention, restraint/side rail elimination, elder mistreatment and legal liability issues. In recognition of her work, she was the 2001 recipient of the Otsuka/American Geriatrics Society Outstanding Scientific Achievement for Clinical Investigation Award. She is a Fellow of the American Academy of Nursing, the Gerontological Society of America, and the New York Academy of Medicine.

William T. Lawson, III, BA, BSA, JD earned his BS (Accounting) and his JD from Villanova University in 1980. He is admitted to practice law in Pennsylvania, New York, and Georgia. He maintains his primary law practice in Philadelphia, with a specialization in nursing home litigation and elder law. Mr. Lawson is a member of the American Association of Justice and is listed in Who's Who in American Law. He provides pro bono legal services for indigent elders through Judicare and Villanova University's law school mentorship program. Mr. Lawson has published and lectured in the areas of nursing home litigation, elder law and elder abuse legislation.

Patricia Iyer, RN, MSN, LNCC is president of The Pat Iyer Group, which provides education for legal nurse consultants at www.legalnursebusiness.com. She assists legal nurse consultants to skyrocket their businesses. Her coaching academy, LNCAcademyinc.com, provides education, support, encouragement and networking opportunities. She has been a legal nurse consultant since 1987 when she first began reviewing cases as an expert witness. She achieved national prominence through her texts and many contributions to the legal nurse consulting field. She was the chief editor of Legal Nurse Consulting Principles and Practices, Second Edition, the core curriculum for legal nurse consulting. She completed 5 years on the Board of Directors of the American Association of Legal Nurse Consultants including a term as president. She was president of a legal nurse consulting business, Med League Support Services, Inc. from 1989 to 2015. She has talked to attorneys about hundreds of claims before providing medical and nursing expert witnesses.

Introduction

This book presents a comprehensive overview of falls as they exist in this country. Falls are a widespread public health problem, affecting many age-groups from children through older adults, from public to patient settings. In the healthcare setting, all persons involved in the delivery of health care- from administration through hands-on healthcare providers and professionals- have a responsibility for providing patient safety and in preventing falls. This shared goal and responsibility for fall prevention (and management) is echoed in the Joint Commission National Patient Safety Standards - affecting all participating hospitals, nursing homes, assisted living facilities, ambulatory care settings or any place where a patient fall can occur. In order to prevent or manage patient falls, whenever and wherever possible, we provide detailed information from our current body of knowledge and understanding, so the reader can decipher if appropriate interventions were in place in at the time a fall occurred.

This text is directed at two audiences - the clinician, and the legal nurse consultant or expert witness. It presents primary interventions for clinicians directed at screening persons at risk for a fall or modifying the "practice" environment to prevent falls and those secondary interventions and is aimed at reducing the reoccurrence of falls. Utilizing this knowledge will help the expert witness designated to testify about the standard of care. The information is also of value to the legal nurse consultant, an individual working as an employee of a law firm, insurance company, or other entity, or as a self-employed consultant. This individual assists legal professionals analyze the most relevant information related to the fall to easily identify related liability or damage/injuries issues. Critical thinking points are highlighted for the legal nurse consultant or clinicians to contemplate related to these key areas.

Overview of Falls in America
by Deanna Gray-Miceli

CHAPTER 1

Chapter 1 Overview of Falls in America
Deanna Gray-Miceli, DNSc, APRN, FAANP

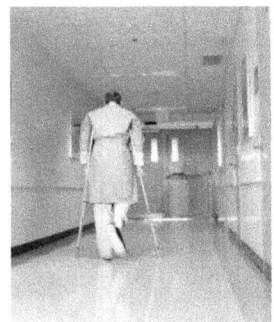

Figure 1.1 Environmental Hazard of a Highly Polished Floor

A. National Imperatives

Falls are a public health problem that has no geographic boundaries or age restrictions. Anyone can fall. Most individuals know of someone, if not themselves, who has fallen. In early childhood years, unless confined in movement or mobility from disease, children fall to the ground quite often, for instance, during childhood play. Some individuals may continue to fall throughout their life and into advancing older years, by virtue of lifelong patterns of clumsiness, "accidentally", from progressive diseases, or from combinations of any or all of these factors. A critical question is: "Does this mean that these falls could have been prevented?" The answer to this question depends on the circumstances of the fall and its likely cause, which can only be answered when the right set of questions is asked and answered.

A fall later in life cannot be categorized as a "normal" event solely because the adult is over age 65; there are many older adults who never experience a fall. Rather, a fall by an older adult could be discerned "abnormal" when other criterion are considered, for instance, the presence of an acute or chronic illness or adverse reaction due to a medication. As a point of comparison, it is assumed that childhood falls are, for the most part, a "normal" part of growth and development. However, incidences occur when falls are not normal, but due to a medical illness, such as a brain tumor or epilepsy.

Falls are a national public health problem because of their magnitude (high incidence), wide scope (affecting all ages, from childhood through older years), and their potentially devastating aftermath (ranging from fatality to serious physical injury or impairment). Fall reduction is a priority. National campaigns have been directed at the two groups at the extremes of the age continuum, the very young (i.e. children) and those over age 65 (older adults). The *National Safety Campaign for Safe Kids* focuses on injury prevention in youth; the *Falls Free* campaign funded by the National Council on Aging focuses on fall and injury prevention among older adults. In both age-groups, falls are the leading cause of unintentional injuries.

When we think about falls and their prevention, what usually comes to mind are individual circumstances of fall events, underlying causes, environmental issues (as shown in Figure 1-1), professional standards of care, and organizational care, such as institutional policies. Falls can occur when organizational systems, due to inadequately trained manpower or insufficient resources, fail to provide acceptable levels of patient care or state of the art interventions for fall prevention. Many systems and organizational failures have been reported in the Institute of Medicine Report, *To Err is Human*.[1] In response, a public policy was created with mandatory requirements for hospitals and/or medical care facilities (nursing homes, assisted living facilities, out-patient surgical centers) to create a culture of patient safety. Nationally, two formidable interventions are recognized, the Patient Safety and Quality Improvement Act of 2005 and the Joint Commission National Patient Safety Goals (NPSGs). The Patient Safety and Quality Improvement Act of 2005 seeks to improve health care delivery through the analysis of medical errors and the recommendation of procedures and processes to minimize future occurrences. The Act establishes a voluntary and confidential structure for providers, including individual professionals and entities, to report information on errors to Patient Safety Organizations.[1] Patient falls are often considered preventable and foreseeable adverse events. Typically falls with injury are reportable under the Patient Safety and Quality Improvement Act of 2005.

The Joint Commission (formerly known as the Joint Commission for Accreditation of Healthcare Organizations) sets the standard for policies, standards and recommended initiatives to shape the delivery of safe health care in the United States. NPSGs drive care in medical care settings such as assisted living facilities, ambulatory care settings, behavioral healthcare, hospitals, disease-specific care centers, home care, laboratories, long-term care and other healthcare organizations. The new National Patient Safety Goals required by all Joint Commission-accredited settings address fall risk assessment of patients and review of existing hospital-wide plans for fall prevention and/or management. The Goals are shown below in Figure 1-2.

Figure 1-2 Joint Commission Fall Prevention Goals

National Patient Safety Goal #9 Falls - Reduce the risk of patient harm resulting from falls.
9A Fall risk- Assess and periodically reassess each patient's risk for falling, including the potential risk associated with the patient's medication regimen, and take action to address any identified risks. *(Retired to the Accreditation Standards)*
9B Fall Reduction Program Implement a fall reduction program and evaluate the effectiveness of the program. [Applicable to Assisted Living, Critical Access Hospital, Disease-Specific Care, Home Care, Hospital, Long Term Care]

On a larger scale, solutions to the problem of falling are also achievable through the Public Health Surveillance (PHS) system. Falls fit into the description of a health-related event of public health importance because they affect many people, require large expenditures of resources, and contain levels of preventability.[2] Falls are systematically monitored, tabulated, and analyzed through administrative and surveillance databanks so that incidence and prevalence trends can be determined, monitored, costs estimated, clinical courses studied, benchmarking performed, and comparative assessments made, such as ratios of disability-adjusted life years (DALYs).[3] DALYs are computations of numerical data expressing the likelihood of life years remaining given the impact or factor of disability. The PHS system plays a major role in not only surveillance and collecting aggregate data about falls and injurious outcomes, but in analyzing trend data so that corrective interventions may be employed. National campaigns exist due largely in part to public awareness garnered through data from PHS surveillance. It was the PHS system that eradicated diseases known to be a communicable and or a threat to one's health. For example, many major health threats such as typhoid, pellagra and goiter, smallpox, heart disease, and infectious diseases were first identified through the PHS system before treatment interventions were devised.[4]

B. Defining Falls

It is important to discuss the definition of falling from both a broad and a narrow focus. From a public health perspective, fall incidence has an enormous scope and magnitude, which has been addressed by governing bodies and national health policy. From a narrower perspective, falls are defined by the people experiencing them, healthcare organizations, where individuals may temporarily or permanently reside, and by professionals, who provide health care to them. Falls were termed "accidents" up until the 1980s. In fact, it was not until the mid-1980s that the term "accidental fall" was replaced by the current and broader term "fall" by the Center for Disease Control (CDC). Given this operational definition of an "accidental fall", interventions were primarily focused on environmental safety. Current knowledge of fall etiology has expanded however, now reinforcing the use of a more general term "fall", which reflects various potential mechanisms of causation and underlying etiologies. Search engines still use the major heading "accidental fall" in describing literary databases about falls.

Figure 1-3 Fall-related Terms

Terms commonly used to describe falls
Accidental fall
Ambulatory fall
Bed-fall
Bi-pedal fall
Chair-fall
Injurious fall
Isolated fall
Near fall
Recurrent fall
Syncopal fall
Trip/slip
True fall
Unintentional-injury related fall
Unwitnessed fall
Witnessed fall

1. Clinical perspective of patient falling

In clinical practice, adjectives used to define patient falls refer to their situational context. For instance, *ambulatory* or what used to be termed "bi-pedal" falls occur while walking or moving, during ambulation. *Bed-falls* occur when patients may slip from the side of the bed or over the side-rail, if used, to a fall to the ground. *Chair-falls* occur either by way of getting out of a chair or getting into (sitting on) a chair. Other adjectives used in clinical practice to define falls may be according to their emergent nature or diagnostic-related type of coding. For example, a *syncopal-fall* conveys a medical emergency associated with a fall, i.e. syncope (a black out or temporary loss of consciousness) occurred precipitating a fall. A listing of various terms describing fall events is presented in Figure 1-3. In clinical practice in a medical care setting, it is important to identify all types of falls.

From a clinical perspective, falls are defined as an "inadvertent landing to the lowest level or ground surface, and not the result of loss of consciousness."[5] In clinical practice settings governed by Centers for Medicare and Medicaid (CMS) such as nursing homes, falls are defined as any event when the resident is found on the floor. CMS regulations state a fall is "unintentionally coming to rest on the ground, floor, or other lower level but not as a result of an overwhelming external force (i.e. being pushed by another patient/resident)." This definition takes into account all falls, witnessed or non-witnessed, when residents are found on the floor. Those eased to the floor or lower level by a caregiver (what would be called a near fall) are also tabulated as having experienced a fall. From an epidemiological stance, when near falls are tabulated as actual "true" falls, incidences are likely to be over-inflated and misrepresented.

Figure 1-4 Two Definitions of Falls

A fall is an inadvertent landing to the lowest level or ground surface, and not the result of loss of consciousness.

A fall is unintentionally coming to rest on the ground, floor, or other lower level but not as a result of an overwhelming external force (i.e. being pushed by another patient/resident.)

From a clinical practice stance, a fall occurring when the patient is eased to the ground could still result in an injury, thus there are legal ramifications from all falls occurring in a medical care setting (See Chapter 6). The CMS definition of this type of fall is broad enough for good reason - so as to make clear that *any and all* events whereby the person ends up on the floor constitutes a fall. Practitioners or facilities may fail to consider this type of fall, as an actual fall (as reflected in their definition of a fall as obtained in the facility policy or procedure manual for fall prevention). Healthcare providers may conceptualize this type of fall as one with which they assisted, therefore, it is not "really" a fall. When an older adult has a diagnosis of osteoporosis, any impact with a hard surface such as the ground or floor or even bed-rail, can potentially produce a break in the already thinned and fragile bone, resulting in a fracture.

If the healthcare provider fails to document this incident as a fall in the medical record because he or she considers it to be an "assisted to the ground" fall, or if an incident report is not completed as required by policy, the only *potential sufferer is the patient*. Unexplained fractures or acute or chronic pain localized to an extremity may indicate that a fall occurred. The failure to record a fall, even though perceived as non-harmful, provides the appearance of a cover up. This may be construed as tampering with the medical record, and significantly increases liability.

Typically cognitively intact patients can recall and report falls. However, a caregiver may recognize signs of injury when a fall is unreported. When the patient cannot provide an explanation, the caregiver should turn to roommates, family members, and other staff to seek an explanation of what may have occurred. Review of documentation tracing back in time from the onset of an unexplained fracture or sudden-acute pain may help isolate other important events that may have occurred.

A fall is coded by its linkage to injury outcomes when a person requires medical attention either by an emergency department or medical care facility. This is done for diagnostic and reimbursement purposes, and also for surveillance purposes when utilized by the PHS. Usually this coding and definition of a fall is according to an external injury classification scheme, hence, the term *E-codes*. This schematic was developed and published for international use by a group of experts, referred to as the International Classification of Diseases (ICD) Handbook.[7] These E-codes typify environmental etiologies of falls as they represent the mechanism of fall occurrence, i.e., in a parking lot, on a slippery sidewalk, off an airplane and so on. Examples of various E-code nomenclatures are presented in Table 1-1.

Table 1-1 Examples of Accidental Falls: (E800-E999 Codes). Reference: International Classification of Diseases (ICD)-9-CM (9th revision). (2001). Los Angeles, CA: Practice Management Information Management.

Falls occurring (in or from):	Assigned E code
Burning building	E890.8
Fall on or from sidewalk curb	E880.1
Fall from chair	E884.2
Fall from bed	E884.4
Unspecified fall	E888.9

Within the PHS domain, falls are further defined according to their linkage to injury outcomes and classified as belonging to either: a) intentional causes, or b) unintentional causes. Intentional falls refer to falls that occur during a suicide or homicide act. Falls are classified as unintentional-injury events across all age groups, (i.e., from birth through 85+ years of age). Also included in this unintentional injury classification are other common injuries resulting from motor vehicle accidents, pedestrian accidents, poisonings, drowning, fires and burns and suffocation. National statistics of injuries due to falls are available for customized reports of injury-related data through the National Center for Injury Prevention and Control (NCIPC).[8]

2. A case definition perspective

Traditionally when a disease-related definition is derived, clear criteria are established serving as a reference point for the diagnosis. Such criteria include histological, morphological and/or pathological changes of cells, tissues, organs or organ systems. In the area of preventable and communicable diseases and other health related problems, case definitions are used as the standard operational definition for which detection, monitoring and tracking are accomplished across administrative and surveillance databanks within the PHS.

> Falling is not a disease of older adults, but considered a clinical condition or geriatric syndrome. There are no laboratory assays or diagnostic tests to reveal fall morphology or pathology.

The case definition of falling defines it as an event, reported or observed or even unwitnessed, but found on the floor, whereby the person lands at the lowest level or ground surface. For example, an environmental fall could be a fall that occurred from a slippery surface. Current International Classification of Diseases definitions links falls to injury outcomes as subclassified through the external "E code nomenclature." Case definitions aside from environmental-related falls are evolving as the science continues to recognize various reasons why different populations of people fall (ranging from medications to acute medical events such as strokes or seizures). National work-groups with representation from the CDC, the State and Territorial Injury Prevention Directors Association (STIPDA) and National Center for Injury Prevention (NCIPC) have recently produced a consensus definition that addresses both injurious and non-injurious types of falls for surveillance purposes.[9] It includes a case definition of falling and fall-related injury outcomes, broad enough to encompass the various mechanisms of fall occurrences (the location or place of fall occurrence) and consequences (the physical injury outcomes), but not the underlying pathological or medically related reason, if any, as to why the fall occurred.

Figure 1-5 Consensus Definition of Falls and Fall-related Injury

A fall is an event which results in the person coming to rest on the ground or other lower level precipitated by a misstep such as a slip, trip or stumble; from loss of grip or balance; from jumping, or from being pushed, bumped, or moved by another person, animal, or inanimate object or force.

A fall-related injury is an injury precipitated by a fall (defined above) and caused by striking an injury-producing surface.

3. The researcher's perspective

Falls are also specifically defined or operationalized by clinical researchers, using adjectives such as "one-time or isolated falls" and "a period of frequent falling or recurrent falling." These fall definitions refer to the frequency of the falls reported per person within a specified period of time. From a research perspective, identification of the fall frequency allows one to analyze and compare similar groups. Falls are defined according to the setting in which they occur, the outcome, and the type of data analyzed. To date, there are no universal case definitions or position statements defining falls and injuries across the multiple databases which analyze falls.

4. The falling person's perspective

All persons who fall have their own unique perceptions and experiences framing how they define a fall. Because of associated myths or pre-conceived beliefs that it is "normal" to fall in old age, older people may actually fall, but call it something else. For instance, a trip or slip may occur and the person falls to the ground, but does not injure himself. When asked if he fell, he may reply "No, I just slipped."

Some older adults who describe their experience of falling have operationalized their own definition of falling according to their view of what it meant. [10] In other instances, the fall may be recalled by the older adult based on the injury sustained.

C. Fall Epidemiology: Magnitude, Scope and Economic Impact

1. Overview of data sources

A glance at the U.S. National Map prepared by WISQARS (Web-based Injury Statistics Query and Reporting System) which reports the leading cause of deaths and injuries illustrates the magnitude of the problem of falling. [11] This data underscore the need for a national imperative to reduce falls. Age-groups (the young and the older adults) experiencing the highest incidences of falls are described in more detail as they are currently tabulated according to *fatal or non-fatal* outcomes. *Incidence* is expressed as the number of new cases reported and *prevalence* is expressed as the number of new and old cases reported. Although the incidence of non-fatal falls is highest among children and older adults, the older adult is more likely to incur a fatal fall.

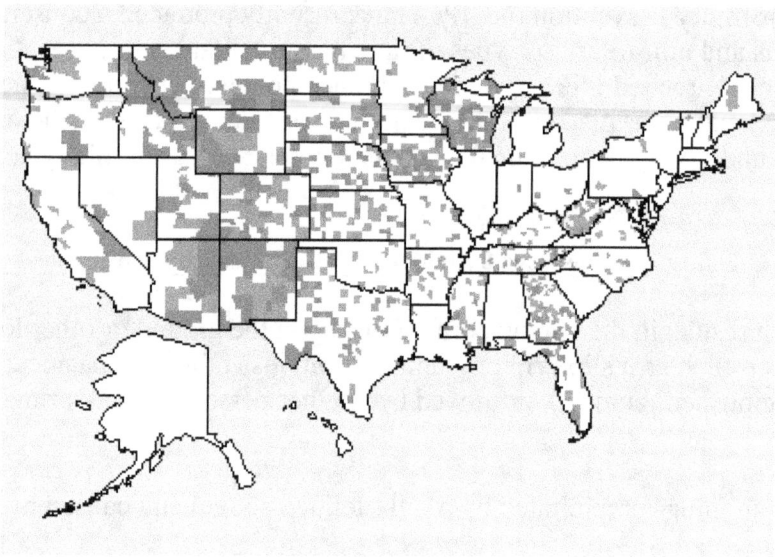

Figure 1-6 WISQARS Falls Mortality Data

2. Fatal fall incidences (children and older adults)

The injury mortality data for unintentional fall deaths per 100,000 is drawn primarily from the vital record or vital statistics data collected by the Center for Disease Control. Vital statistics record information about the health of a population, such as the total number of live births, deaths due to cancer, and so on. Falls are sub-coded due to the mechanism of injury, using ICD-10 codes.

The vital record data provide the only virtually complete reporting source for injury fatality. [12]

Falls are particularly harmful to children. Unintentional injury (all types) causes almost 40 percent of deaths among infants and children to age 4 years. [13] Each year, an average of 2 children die due to baby-walker related injuries. [14] During 1990-2000, the National Center for Injury Prevention and

Control reported that 147 children aged 14 and younger died from playground related injuries. Twenty percent died from falls to the playground surface; most of the deaths occurred on home playgrounds.[15]

Fatalities occurred when children fell from great heights (greater than 2 stories or 6.7 m [22 feet]), or when the head of a child hit a hard surface such as concrete.[16] Each year, about 18 children ages 10 and under die from window-related injuries.[17] From age one through ages 85+ the number of fatal falls steadily rises over the years and then reaches a high peak at age 70+, continuing to rise for those 85+. In 2002, there were 53 deaths per 100,000 persons for all sexes and races among newborn to 4 years old. In this same year, there were 1,208 deaths per 100,000 for those age 70-74, 2,011 deaths per 100,000 for those 75-79 years of age, and 5,990 per 100,000 for those age 85+. Nationwide, falls rank as the eighth leading cause of unintentional injury deaths among adults over age 65.[18] "The State of Home Safety in America" study highlights the magnitude of fall-related unintentional home injury deaths, accounting for 49 percent of deaths for adults aged 60 to 69, and 66 percent of the deaths for adults greater than 70 years of age.[19] The Traumatic Brain Injury (TBI) registries also highlight serious outcomes of falls, as they are a leading cause of TBI among *all* age groups.

Critical thinking point for the clinician or legal nurse consultant: Was the person who fell at high risk for a fatal fall based on age? Did the plan of care address this concern or was there routine use of the same plan of care for all falling persons irrespective of age or injury?

While interventions for the prevention of falls and associated injuries and fatalities must be individualized to the person and their unique circumstances, the type of intervention chosen is also contingent upon the current state of the science of effective (empirically tested) interventions. According to the most current reported incidence of fatal falls in the United States, adults over age 85 have the highest risk of fatality due to an unintentional fall.

3. Non-fatal fall incidences and injuries (children and older adults)

Falls contribute greatly to morbidity and mortality. Falls among children are the leading cause of hospitalizations; sports injuries are the leading cause of emergency department visits.[20] More than 12 million nonfatal falls in homes per year result in injuries necessitating medical care.[21] Nearly 4 million emergency department visits and 4.2 million office-based physician visits were made because of a fall in 1999, and over 2,145,044 people lost at least one day from work or school due to falls.[22]

National estimates of non-fatal injuries are reported by United States hospital emergency departments. This represents community dwelling persons who sought medical care. Data are coded using E-codes from the ICD nomenclature. Of the top 10 leading causes of non-fatal injury in the United States, for all races and sexes in 2004, the *unintentional fall* ranks first in these age groups:

- less than 1 year,
- 1-4 years of age,
- 5-9 years of age,
- 10-14 years of age,
- 25-34 year-olds,
- 35-44 year-olds,
- 45-54 year-olds,
- 55-64 year-old,
- 65-74 year-olds, and
- 85+.[23]

As an example of the magnitude of unintentional falls, in 2004, there were over 1 million infants and children up to age 4 years seen in the emergency room for non-fatal injuries and about one-half million persons over age 85+ seen for unintentional fall injuries. [24] Common sites for falls among children in public places include playgrounds, roadways while bicycle riding, and during contact athletic sports. In the home, falls and deaths from these falls occur from baby-walker related injuries where the majority under age 15 months sustain injuries falling down the steps (76 percent). Nearly 80 percent of infants who suffer injuries are being supervised at the time of the incident and the caregiver is present in the same room as the child. [25] Falls often occur from cribs, beds and furniture, bathtubs and particularly windows. The majority of window related deaths (70 percent) occur during the spring and summer months among boys under age 5 who are unsupervised. Window-related falls tend to occur in large, urban areas, low-income neighborhoods such as children living in apartment buildings. [26] The National Safe Kids campaign addresses common hazards and their prevention in an effort to reduce the total number of falls, particularly falls associated with fatality and injury.

4. Fatal fall incidence in the workplace

Fall related injuries and deaths occurring in the workplace are events we care not to think about. But each day, men and women who perform "high risk" jobs are at high risk for falls and fatal injuries if they fail to follow proper safety precautions or if their equipment fails. According to the National Institute for Occupational Safety and Health (NIOSH), falls are the leading cause of traumatic occupational death. Over a five year period, 3,491 persons fell to their death while working and 17 percent fell from a scaffold. [27] Falls may occur from cranes, construction sites, roofs, and other high places. Investigation has found that it is the suspension scaffold that is most dangerous.

5. Economic impact of falls

The estimated economic costs of injuries sustained in the home due to falls rank the highest compared to other injuries like burns, suffocation, and poisonings and totaled over $90 billion in 1998. [28] Besides physical injury, direct costs and loss of work, serious falls often change lives forever among older individuals. [29] A recent report compiled by the U.S. Consumer Product Safety Commission (CPSC) from 1991-2002 and Neighborhood Safety Network, entitled "Emergency Room Injuries for Adults 65 and Older", draws attention to the percentage increase of adults 75 years and older entering U.S. hospital emergency rooms with consumer product-related injuries. [30] They report adults age 75 and older have twice the rate of emergency room treated injuries associated with consumer products compared to those 65-74. Over three-quarters (77 percent) of these emergency room visits involved falls. This report also compiled typical fall scenarios. (For more detail see Chapter 2).

In 2002, there were 85,630 emergency-treated injuries and 220,630 medically treated injuries that specifically occurred in the bathroom. Twenty-seven percent of these people were hospitalized; 194 died with overall injury costs estimated at over $6 million dollars and $970 million in death costs. [31]

Treatment for fall-related injuries accounts for a disproportionately high use and expenditure of health care resources in the elderly. One study estimates that the average cost for a fall-related hospitalization in 1996 was $11,042, with nursing home costs of $5,325, and total health-related costs of $19,440. [32] Aside from the obvious serious physical effects and/or damages, falls can have devastating psychological effects which impact on quality of life.

Fear of subsequent falls may lead to self-imposed limitation of activities and result in confinement inside one's home and feelings of isolation, helplessness and or loss. The economic impact of all of the factors influencing mental health has yet to be fully determined in the overall health-related costs for self-imposed limitation of activities due to falls. .

6. Overview of the incidence of falls in medical care settings

Falls may occur anywhere: adult and pediatric day care, general acute care hospitals, assisted living facilities which provide medical and professional nursing care, skilled nursing units, clinics, dialysis units, nursing homes and specialized children's hospitals. Many falls in these settings require emergency department care and hospitalization depending on the type and severity of injury. Some may result in litigation. To date, although patient safety laws (adopted by some states) require medical care facilities to report all adverse events due to preventable fall incidences, there is no centralized aggregate incidence of fall data from United States hospitals, other than falls with injury.

Although aggregate injurious fall data are known and coded by external injury causes (E-codes), those "unspecified" falls *without injury* are not routinely coded, reported or analyzed according to their linkage to antecedent events in hospital settings. From a public policy and clinical practice stance, this potentially jeopardizes both the projection of services needed for patients and the clinical management thereof. Allocation of services to meet the healthcare needs of people cannot be projected when actual numbers of falls are not uniformly reported. Further, a change in the clinical management and policies and procedures is warranted when persons are falling *once* versus *repeatedly*. Interventions geared toward primary and secondary prevention can be better addressed should a national databank or injury state surveillance systems become available.

a. Falls in the nursing home

Although only a relatively small percentage of older Americans reside in long-term care institutions in this country, many older adults transition in and out of these settings during periods of recovery from illness. To date, there are about 1.63 million older adults residing in nursing homes nationwide; of these, nearly 75 percent experience a fall each year.[33] It has been estimated that nearly 40 percent of patients will fall again. Most falls in nursing homes are non-witnessed; when residents who suffer from dementia cannot recall the circumstances, there is speculation as to if and how a fall occurred. Oftentimes fall events are simply categorized as "found on floor." Up to 50 percent of nursing home residents fall each year, which is two to three times that of community-dwelling residents.[34, 35, 36] Among those with Alzheimer's disease or other dementing illnesses, the annual incidence of falls is twice the rate of older persons without dementia.[37]

Critical thinking point for the clinician or legal nurse consultant: What mechanisms are in place to identify, tabulate and trend fall occurrences and potential falls with injury occurrences in nursing homes on a routine basis (for instance, every shift, daily and/or monthly?) What are the procedures for fall monitoring when the same older patient falls repeatedly in a short period of time? Does the staff receive feedback on the incidence of falls on their nursing unit, and what they can be doing to make the environment safer?

It has been estimated that with the aging of the baby boomers there will be a 25.8 percent increase in injurious falls between 1995-2020 resulting in more than 17 million injurious falls by 2020.[38]

b. Falls in children's hospitals

Although national incidences of pediatric falls in hospital settings are difficult to obtain and not available at the time of this writing, younger patients do experience falls in these facilities during illness treatment or recovery. Children may fall from bed or while ambulating or running on the unit. The facility staff needs to be aware of children at higher risk to fall or sustain injury such as those with uncontrolled epilepsy, those with fragile bones susceptible to extremity fracture, or children with hemopoetic disorder predisposed to bleeding disorders. With the new Joint Commission standards for patient safety, facilities will be required to monitor the incidence and trends of falling among hospitalized children as well as for adults.

c. Falls in acute care-hospitals

State departments of health that analyze patient safety data have reported to Joint Commission up to 30 percent of adverse medical events are due to patient falls. Fall incidence data linked to injury outcome is aggregately available within individual state departments of health. This data may have additional information such as place of fall occurrence (emergency department, hospital, long-term care facilities transferring to the emergency department and so on). At present, other than from individual states, there are no centralized, national fall statistics for "falls without injury" events occurring in general hospitals (a place of occurrence). Tabulated fall data is for "fall with injury". The Agency for Health Care Quality and Research (AHRQ) reported that general hospitals experience on average one million falls among hospitalized persons. Joint Commission reports an increase in adverse medical events due to patient falls from 2.6 percent in 2002 to 5.2 percent in 2006. [39] Given the magnitude of falls in this setting, it is expected that additional surveillance and trend analysis methods will need to be developed in order to capture aggregate fall incidence. Hip fracture is one of the patient safety indicators measured by AHRQ in hospitalized populations. Although the rate of hospitalizations for hip fractures decreased during 2001-2005 [40], hip fracture injury contributes substantially to mortality and morbidity among older adults.

D. Consequences of Falls

1. Overview of common injuries

Despite the high incidence of falls among older adults, most falls in this age group do not result in physical injury. Fall-related injuries seen among older age groups include all fractures, other serious injuries (dislocated joints, subdural or subarachnoid hematomas, lacerations requiring sutures, and soft tissue injuries requiring medical treatment), and minor injuries (lacerations without sutures, bruises, abrasions, certain sprains, and other soft tissue injuries). An overall higher rate of both falls and fall-related injuries occurs among the elderly, especially among those with dementia. [41]

Critical thinking point for the clinician or legal nurse consultant: What might you look for in the medical record of a patient who fell and was unable to accurately verify what happened because of aphasia, young or old age, critical illness, amnesia or dementia? What type of assessment should be done by clinical staff?

There are some signs and symptoms that a clinician typically looks for that are indicative of a potential problem following an injury. These include:

- a change in behavior or function that is different–for instance, an ambulatory person suddenly cannot weight bear or stops walking altogether;
- pain - the person holds a body part such as a leg while walking or holds onto the shoulder when reaching for an object and there is no other medical explanation for this change;
- a change in level of consciousness - the person was always alert and oriented; now he or she is sleepy all the time and disoriented.

2. Hip fracture

Approximately 11 percent (range 1 to 36 percent) of falls in nursing homes result in injury; hip fractures account for 1 to 6 percent of fall-related injuries in nursing home residents.[42] More than 90 percent of hip fractures result from falls, with the great majority occurring in those over the age of seventy.[43] Fractures other than of the hip or pelvis account for about 2 to 3 percent of fall-related injuries[44] while serious soft tissue injuries requiring medical intervention and causing impaired functional status represent approximately 10 percent of falls.[45] Almost half of hospitalizations for trauma were fall-related in women 85 years of age and older (who represent the average nursing home resident).[46] In fact, the Centers for Disease Control and Prevention (CDC) reports that from 1988 to 1996, women 85 years and older were almost 8 times more likely than women 65-74 years old to be hospitalized for fall-related hip fractures.[47] CDC data analysis also shows that older white women suffer from hip fractures at much higher rates than older white men, black men, or black women. This is thought to be partially due to the higher prevalence of osteoporosis among older white women, a condition that contributes to a reduction in bone mass, increased bone fragility, and leads to fractures after minimal trauma.[48] There were over 321,000 hospital admissions from hip fracture in 2000, a number projected to exceed 500,000 by 2040.[49] Hip fracture is a serious consequence of osteoporosis and constitutes a major public health problem worldwide.[50]

Figure 1-7 Examples of Injuries from Non-fatal Falls

Physical Injury
- Hip fracture
- Pelvic fracture
- Vertebral fracture
- Wrist fracture
- Subdural hematoma (SDH)
- Traumatic brain injury (TBI)
- Rhabdomyolitis
- Laceration
- Abrasion
- Skin Tear
- Sprain
- Strain
- Contusion

Psychological Injury
- Fear of falling
- Frightfulness
- Helplessness
- Hopelessness

Other types of trauma
- Loss of independence
- Reduced mobility or immobility
- Changed life

Injurious falls are significant because of their role in morbidity and mortality in the elderly. The incidence of falls with hip fracture in the acute care hospital setting is tabulated through external injury codes and then reported in national data banks. As one of twenty Patient Safety Indicators [PSI] monitored, post-operative hip fracture occurred among 5,200 in-patients in 2000, and the risk for this PSI increased with age.[51] Despite sophisticated surgical procedures for hip fracture repair, it has been well established that older adults suffer substantial decline in physical functioning (ability to dress, transfer from bed to chair, walk, climb stairs) after hip fracture.[52] Half of those people over 75 who suffer a fall-related hip fracture will die within one year of the fall.[53] In fact, one recent study found hip fracture mortality to range between 10 percent to 28 percent at 6 months.[54] An individual's post-surgery recovery is dependent on co-morbid conditions (other medical illnesses) and level of dependency prior to the fracture[55]; consequently, nursing home residents may require longer rehabilitation and are the least likely to do well after suffering a hip fracture. Morbidity and mortality statistics related to falls verify the need for increased prevention efforts.

Fall-related *serious* injury, especially hip fracture, is associated with significant mortality rates.[51] Those with hip fractures have a 17 to 33 percent mortality rate within one year, and 25 to 33 percent become severely disabled or unable to walk after one year.[56, 57] Mortality rates and severity of complications from hip fracture also sharply rises with increasing age.[58, 59]

3. Traumatic brain injury

Traumatic brain injury [TBI] is another serious injurious outcome of falls. Of the 50,000 deaths from traumatic brain injury, falls are the leading cause among those 75 and older.[60] Children also sustain traumatic brain injuries. This is one factor driving the National Safe Kids campaign for fall and injury prevention.

4. Psychological injury

Although a major fracture or head trauma is considered a serious injury, older adults may define lesser trauma as "serious" which relates to their unique perceptions and personal experiences of a fall. A community-based sample of older adults defined "a serious fall" as one that changed their lives by confinement, feeling helpless, frustrated and/or unable to do the things they normally did."[61] These accounts are likely to be reflective of social issues such as the personal loss of prestige or even stigmata of what the fall signified. Fear of falling is reported in the geriatric literature as a major psychological after-effect of falling.[62] It has been observed in both non-falling and falling older adults. Figure 1-7 illustrates a composite picture of the types of physical and psychological aftermath or trauma encompassing the experience of a non-fatal fall. Fear that an elder may fall may limit the staff's efforts to encourage ambulation. When the staff is overprotective, the patients' fear of falling may increase, with resultant reluctance to push themselves to be active. This may lead to a more sedentary activity level than desirable.

Critical thinking point for the pediatric clinician or legal nurse consultant: Are there institutional policies or interventions for children deemed at greatest risk for head injury? Is protective head gear available? Are there policies or interventions related to protecting extremities from fracture in susceptible at risk children? How might the immediate plan of care be different if the patient is thought to have incurred a TBI post-fall?

Critical thinking point for the clinician or legal nurse consultant: Other than verbal statement from the resident, what types of routine information collected during a resident's stay in a facility might identify or verify the impact a fall has had on an older adult's life?

One might look to the patient's baseline capabilities–in terms of functional status - as noted on admission to a facility through the MDS (Minimum Data Set- a standardized admission assessment used in nursing homes.) For example, the resident was able to walk unassisted before a fall. Following the fall, the patient may need a wheelchair for mobility. While this is commonly assumed to be because of some physical injury, in the absence of physical injury, one should consider psychological injury such as fear of falling and/or walking. There is a range of possible expressions and actions by older patients that may be indicative of a reluctance to regain previous lifestyle due to fear to ambulate (see Figure 1-8 for statements of older adults' experiences of a serious fall.)

It is important for nursing staff to assess the older patient/resident for fear of falling, especially following a fall. Questions asked to cognitively intact people should be directed toward identifying fear of falling, which might limit their lifestyle. Older adult patients can be helped through individual counseling and other behavioral techniques to reduce fear of falling.

E. Patterns of Falls and Their Significance

Although falls can occur for a multitude of reasons, it is recognition of pattern(s) that is most helpful to practitioners. The patient and the primary care practitioner are in the best position to decipher the patterns.

Should a patient continuously fall, the practitioner must question why this is happening. While persons may fall only once, in an *isolated* fashion, it is the person who falls *repeatedly* who is of greater concern. Sometimes, when a person falls repeatedly, the practitioner may actually expect it, given the patient's medical history, prognosis, or use of certain medication associated with falling. In some cases, repeated falling is consistent with underlying medical problems (and a natural progression of disease pathology), as in the case of Parkinson's disease. In other cases, repeatedly falling is not expected and indeed associated with preventable medical events, circumstances, and medications.

When clients (whether they are young children or older adults) fall in a medical care setting, it is the responsibility of the primary practitioner to determine the underlying etiology and to put into place a plan of care that addresses known risks and potential underlying causes in order to prevent future falls. Furthermore, during a comprehensive fall evaluation, it is expected that certain questions are asked and examinations take place (according to standards of practice for fall evaluation). Typically a geriatric specialist is capable of such evaluation. In practice, clinicians consult national recommendations or clinical practice guidelines developed by experts. These guidelines give some direction to the content to include in a fall assessment, but not necessarily the exact questions, leaving some discretion to the practitioner. Because of the serious aftermath of falls and associated complications like hip fracture, national and professional organizations serving the elderly have formulated guidelines for fall prevention (see Chapter 3 for more detail).

This chapter has presented an overview of magnitude, scope and impact of falls within America across public and healthcare settings. The prevention of falls depends on detecting why they occur and minimizing risks associated with falls. The following chapter addresses why falls occur in the first place, which lays the foundation for an understanding of the types of interventions chosen for fall and injury prevention.

Figure 1-8 Descriptions of Older Adults' Most Serious Fall

A 67-year-old woman: "I was incapacitated for weeks, at least, and it (the fall) is still hampering what I can do."

An 84-year-old woman: "The horror was when the bruises formed. I would not go out until they were mostly cleared away. I had a face you could frighten children with."

An 86-year-old woman: "I felt like a kid, calling 'Mother, help me.'"

An 80-year-old man: "I thought …What am I going to do? I am all alone (laying on the pavement in a parking lot) and I am scared to death. I had great, great frightfulness for all time sake…"

An 84-year-old woman: "I have a fear of falling and I am reluctant to walk when I go out of the apartment by myself; I would take my husband's arm and not just in affection, but in desperation, you know, to hold me up."

Reference: Gray-Miceli, Deanna Lynn (2001). Changed life: A phenomenological study of the meaning of serious falls to older adults (Doctoral dissertation, Widener University, 2001, Chairperson Dr. Barbara Patterson). UMI DissertationAbstracts. (UMI Microform No. 3005877).

EndNotes

[1] Institute of Medicine Report. *To Err is Human; Building a Safer Health System*. National Academy Press, Washington, 2001.

[2] *Legal Basics for Professional Nursing Practice*, Center for American Nurses, 2005.

[3] "Updated Guidelines for Evaluating Public Health Surveillance Systems. Centers for Disease Control and Prevention", *Morbidity and Mortality Weekly Report (MMWR)*, July 27, 2001/50 (RR13). [Online]. Available on Internet at: http://www.cdc.gov/mmwr/preview/mmwrhtml/rr5013a1.htm. Accessed March 28, 2006.

[4] Id.

[5] "MMWR Achievements in Public Health, 1900-1999: Changes in the Public Health System. Centers for Disease Control and Prevention": 48, pgs. 1141-1147, 1999. *The Journal of the American Medical Association (JAMA)* 283, pgs. 735-738, 2000.

[6] Isaacs, B. "Falling all over the place." *Practitioner 231* (8): pgs. 103-107, 1987.

[7] *International Classification of Diseases, 9th Revision, Clinical Modification* Sixth Edition, Millennium Edition (2001). Practice Management Information Corporation.

[8] National Center for Injury Prevention and Control (NCIPC) [Online]. Available on Internet at: http://www.cdc.gov/ncipc/ Accessed March 15, 2006.

[9] State and Territorial Injury Prevention Directors Association (STIPDA), Injury Surveillance Workgroup on Falls [ISW4]Report: Consensus Recommendations for Surveillance of Falls and Fall- related Injuries. Available on the Internet at: http://www.stipda.org/associations/5805/files/ISW4_Report_Final.pdf.

[10] Gray-Miceli, D. L. "Changed life: A phenomenological study of the meaning of serious falls to older adults." [doctoral dissertation]. Chester, PA: Widener University, 2001. *UMI Dissertation Abstracts* (UMI No. 30005877).

[11] Centers for Disease Control and Prevention. Web-based Injury Statistics Query and Reporting System (WISQARS) [Online] (2003). National Center for Injury Prevention and Control. Available at: http://www.cdc.gov/ncipc/wisqars/. Accessed October 3, 2005.

[12] See note 8.

[13] Smith, S.M., Luallen, J.J., Froehlke, RG., & Rodriguez, J.G. "From Data to Action. CDC's Public Health Surveillance for women, infants, and children." [Online]. Available on Internet: http://www.cdc.gov/reproductivehealth/Products&Pubs/DatatoAction/pdf/chlt4.pdf. Accessed March 13, 2006.

[14] National SAFE KIDS Campaign, Injury Fact Sheet, Washington, DC. Available on the Internet at: http://www.usa.safekids.org/tier3_cd.cfm?folder_id=540&content_item_id=1050.

[15] See note 8.

[16] American Academy of Pediatrics Policy Statement. *Pediatrics* 107:5, 1188-1191, May 2001.

[17] See note 14.

[18] See note 11.

[19] Runyan, C. W., Casteel, C., Pekis, D., Black, C., Marshall, S. W., et al. "Unintentional injuries in the homes in the United States. Part I: Mortality." *American Journal of Preventive Medicine,* 28(1), pgs. 73-79, 2005.

[20] Guyer, B., Ellers, B. "Childhood injuries in the United States: mortality, morbidity, and cost." *American Journal of Diseases in Children* 144: pgs. 649-52, 1990.

[21] Runyon, C. W., Perkis, D., Marshall, S. W., Johnson, R.M., Coyne-Beasley, T., et al. "Unintentional injuries in the home environment in the United States. Part II: Morbidity." *American Journal of Preventive Medicine,* 28: pgs. 80-87, 2005.

[22] *International Classification of Diseases (ICD)-9-CM* (9th revision). Los Angeles, CA: Practice Management Information Management. 2001.

[23] See note 8.

[24] Id.

[25] See note 14.

[26] Id.

[27] National Institute of Occupational Safety and Health. Available on the Internet at: //www.cdc.gov/niosh/injury/traumafall.html. Accessed March 31, 2007.

[28] See note 22.

[29] See note 10.

[30] U.S. Consumer Product Safety Commission. "Emergency Room Injuries for Adults 65 and Older". [Online]. Available from Internet: http://www.nsc.org/news/nr02145.htm.

[31] U.S. Preventive Services Task Force *Guide to Clinical Preventive Services: Report of the US Preventive Services Task Force.* 2nd edition (pp.659-685). Baltimore: Williams & Wilkins, 1996.

[32] Rizzo, J. A., Friedkin, R., Williams, C. S., Nabors, J., Acampora, D., & Tinetti, M. E. "Health care utilization and costs in a Medicare population by fall status." *Medical Care,* 36, pgs. 1174-1188, 1998.

[33] See note 8.

[34] Kerse, N., Butler, M., Robinson, E., & Todd, M. "Fall prevention in residential care: a cluster, randomized, controlled trial." *Journal of the American Geriatrics Society,* 52, pgs. 524-531, 2004.

[35] Braun, J. A., & Capezuti, E. A. "The legal and medical aspects of physical restraints and bed side rails and their relationship to falls and fall-related injuries in nursing homes." *DePaul Journal of Healthcare Law,* 4, pgs.1-72, 2000.

[36] Kiely, D. K., Kiel, D. P., Burrows, A., & Lipsitz, L. A. "Identifying nursing home residents at risk for falling." *Journal of the American Geriatrics Society,* 46, pgs. 551-555, 1998.

[37] Capezuti, E., & Talerico, K. A. "Review article: Physical restraint removal and falls and injuries." *Research and Practice in Alzheimer's Disease,* 2, pgs. 338-355, 1999.

[38] Englander, F., Hodson, T. J., & Terregrossa, R. A. "Economic dimensions of slip and fall injuries." *Journal of Forensic Sciences,* 41, pgs. 733-746, 1996.

[39] Joint Commission Sentinel Events 2006. Available on the Internet at: http://www.jcaho.org. Accessed March 31, 2007.

[40] CDC, *Morbidity and Mortality Weekly Report,* November 17, 2006 Vol 55: No. 45.

[41] Rubenstein, L. Z. "Preventing falls in the nursing home." *Journal of the American Medical Association,* 278, pgs. 595-598, 1997.

[42] Cali, C. M., & Kiel, D.P. "An epidemiologic study of fall-related fractures among institutionalized older people." *Journal of the American Geriatrics Society, 43*, pgs.1336-1340, 1995.

[43] Sattin, R. W. "Falls among older persons: A public health perspective." *Annual Review of Public Health,* 13, 489-508, 1992.

[44] Neufeld, R.R., Tideiksaar, R., Yew, E., Brooks, F., Young, J., Browne, G., & Hsu, M.A. "A multidisciplinary falls consultation service in a nursing home." *Gerontologist, 31*, pgs. 120-123, 1991.

[45] Tinetti, M. E. "Instability and falling in elderly patients." *Seminars in Neurology, 9* (1), pgs. 39-45, 1989.

[46] Alexander, B.H., Rivara, F.P., and Wolf, M.E. "The cost and frequency of hospitalization for fall-related injuries in older adults." *American Journal of Public Health*, 82 , pgs. 1020-1023, 1992.

[47] Stevens, J. A., Hasbrouck, L., Durant, T. M., Dellinger, A. M., Batabyal, P. K., Crosby, A. E., et al. "Surveillance for Injuries and Violence Among Older Adults." In: *CDC Surveillance Summaries*, December 17, 1999. MMWR 48 (No. SS-8), pgs. 27-50, 1999.

[48] Id.

[49] Department of Health and Human Services, Health Care Financing Administration. *Medicare State Operations Manual Provider Certification.* Appendix PP: Guidance to surveyors- long term care facilities, October 10, 2000. Retrieved May 28, 2004 from http://www.cms.hhs.gov/manuals/pm_trans/R20SOM.pdf

[50] Melton, L.J. III. 1996. "Epidemiology of hip fractures: implications of the exponential increase with age". *Bone,* 18 (3 Suppl): 121S-125S.

[51] Romano, P.S., Geppert, J.J., Davies, S., Miller, M.R., Elixhauser, A., McDonald, K., 2003. "A national profile of patient safety in U.S. hospitals". *Health Affairs,* 22:2, 154-166.

[52] Young, Y., German, P., Brant, L., et al "The predictors of surgical procedure and the effects of functional recovery in elderly with subcapital fractures." *Journal of Gerontology: Medical Sciences*, 51A, pgs. M158-M164, 1996.

[53] Rawnsky, E. "Review of the literature on falls among the elderly." *Image: Journal of Nursing Scholarship*, 30, pgs. 47-52, 1998.

[54] Keene, G.S., Parker, M.J., Pryor, G.A. "Mortality and morbidity after hip fracture". *British Medical Journal,* 1993:307:1248-50.

[55] Sartoretti, C., Sartoretti-Schefer, S., Ruckert, R., et al. "Comorbid conditions in old patients with femur fractures." *The Journal of Trauma: Injury, Infection and Critical Care, 43,* pgs. 570-577, 1997.

[56] Van Schoor, N. M., Deville, W. L., Bouter, L. M., & Lips, P. "Acceptance and compliance with external hip protectors: a systematic review of the literature." *Osteoporosis International,* 13*,* pgs. 917-924, 2002.

[57] Mgaziner, J., Hawkes, W., Hebel, J. R., Zimmerman, S. I., Fox, K. M., Dolan, M., et al. "Recovery from hip fractures in eight areas of function." *Journal of Gerontology Series A: Biological Sciences and Medical Sciences, 55A, pgs.* M498-M507, 2000.

[58] Roberts, S. E., & Goldacre, M. J. "Time trends and demography of mortality after fractured neck of femur in an English population", 1968-98: database study. *British Medical Journal,* 327*, pgs.* 771, 2003.

[59] Chang, J. T., Morton, S. C., Rubenstein, L. Z., Mojica, W. A., Maglione, M., Suttorp, M. J., et al. "Interventions for the prevention of falls in older adults: systematic review and meta-analysis of randomized clinical trials." *British Medical Journal*, 328, pgs. 680-683, 2004.

[60] Adekoya, N., Thurman, D. J., White, D. D., & Webb, K. W. "Surveillance for traumatic brain injury deaths—United States, 1989-1998." *MMWR Surveillance Summaries,* 51(10), pgs. 1-14, 2002.

[61] See Note 8.

[62] Lach, H.W. "Incidence and risk factors for developing fear of falling in older adults." *Public Health Nursing,* Jan-Feb 22 (1): pgs. 45-52, 2005.

CHAPTER 2

The Multifactorial Nature of Falls
by Deanna Gray-Miceli

Chapter 2 The Multifactorial Nature of Falls
Deanna Gray-Miceli, DNSc, APRN, FAANP

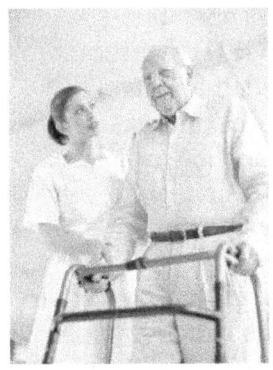

A. Factors Associated with Falls
Falling to the ground can be caused by one of many factors, which may or may not occur simultaneously to produce a fall. At any age, falls can occur because of environmental hazards, adverse side effects from medications, medical reasons, or equipment or device failure, such as unstable furniture. Sometimes the underlying causative agent for a fall is not known despite medical evaluation; falls occurring for these reasons are called idiopathic (not known) or due to happenstance. In older adults, age-related changes may be implicated in falls as well. [1]

Falls are often caused by the interaction of several factors. These factors can be categorized as *intrinsic* (involving the person, ranging from age-related changes to medical diseases) or extrinsic (external to the person involving the environment, situational context and other socio-economic factors.) [2] It is important to identify the risks associated with falling. Tinetti's seminal work in this area found that 27 percent of community dwelling older adults with no-or-only one risk factors, had a fall versus nearly three-quarters of the sample who fell when four or more risk factors were present. [3]

People are at risk for falling when there is a hazardous environment containing uneven pavement, ice, spills, improperly installed or absent handrails, poorly lit stairs, lack of contrast between stairs and the floor, and other factors. Healthcare consumers can be educated about various environmental hazards and how to prevent falls in public places, in the home, assisted living, or in their hospital or nursing home room.

B. Indoor and Outdoor Public Environmental Hazards and Falls
Falls occur in public places such as in stores, on playgrounds, in community neighborhoods, in the workplace, or off ladders and scaffolds. Typically these falls are associated with an unforeseen *environmental* hazard such as an uneven surface, a wet slippery area or inadequate support. In the community, curbs (see Figure 2-1) and playgrounds are maintained by local townships and roadways are maintained by the state department of transportation (DOT). In residential neighborhoods, however, homeowners are responsible for maintaining safe environmental conditions of publicly used walkways or steps. Routine inspection and reporting of hazardous environmental conditions is everyone's responsibility.

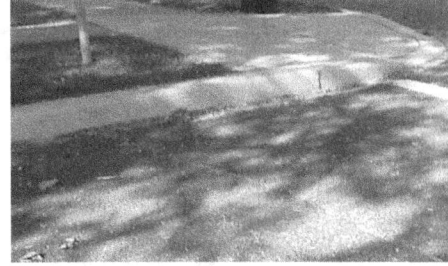

Figure 2-1 Brightly painted curb

Curbs and steps have changes in surface height or depth, which can lead to a fall for individuals with certain predisposed conditions. Use of bright bold color on surface edges such as the curb in figure 2-1 serves as a preventive fall measure. It helps pedestrians who might be visually impaired or suffer from conditions predisposing them to impairments in depth perception. (See section G of this chapter on advancing age for more detail).

Uneven surface edges such as bricks or concrete create instability when walking (see Figure 2-2). This surface may create difficulty and lead to falls for the person with pre-existing difficulty with walking. Foot problems or conditions causing difficulty with walking or balance increase the risk of falls.

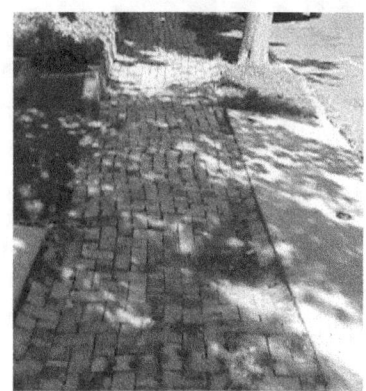

Figure 2-2 Uneven, Dangerous, Sidewalk

In the workplace environment, it is the responsibility of facility management to assess and correct foreseeable hazards which have been reported to involve slips or falls and other types of injury litigation. Depending on the facility size, management may also be required to follow workplace environmental safety rules and regulations according to the Occupational Safety and Health Administration (OSHA). The Public Employees Occupational Safety and Health Program (PEOSH) oversees primary and secondary levels of initiatives for fall prevention for state public employees. Investigations of reported fall occurrences, injuries and fatalities are conducted by administrative officials in the public workplace. They are responsible for providing proactive primary and secondary levels of prevention.

Slips and falls occur frequently in public places and are a common source of litigation. The tort of negligence is dependent on the concept of "foreseeability". If harm is planned, or intended, then it might be considered an intentional tort or even a crime. On the other hand, there is no liability if the fall is an unavoidable accident. However, failing to provide a safe environment often results in a poor outcome, which could be foreseeable. For example, a landlord is expected to provide adequate lighting in stairwells so that individuals will not injure themselves. It is foreseeable that an accident could occur if the lights burn out and are not replaced.

In public places, falls can occur due to slippery surfaces. The personnel of the business are accountable to make sure that the spill is cleaned up in a timely manner, so as to avoid an accidental hazard. Video surveillance, housekeeping records in the form of checklists, or timed logs can be produced to verify surface conditions, the length of time the spill was present, and the extent to which facility management diligently took corrective action to remedy the problem. The evidence may either validate or invalidate the fall victim's statements. For example, surveillance cameras in casinos have caught patrons deliberately spilling water on a floor, faking a fall, and then seeking to be compensated for the so called negligence of the casino.

C. Environmental Hazards in and Around the Home and Their Assessment

Environmental hazards that can lead to falling can be found in and out of doors. These hazards are so common that the National Center for Injury Prevention, Centers for Disease Control produces a consumer pamphlet entitled "Home Safety Checklist". See Appendix One. Use of this checklist by consumers proactively can help to prevent a fall or injury from occurring. Hazards in the home producing falls and associated injury have been potentially problematic for older adults.

The Consumer Product Safety Commission (CPSC) and Neighborhood Safety Network Report (1991-2002) entitled "Emergency Room Injuries for Adults 65 and Older" found that falls and associated injuries were from consumer products that involved:

- the steps,
- transitioning from standing to sitting on furniture,
- the bed,
- the bathtub and/or toilet,
- tripping over telephone cords or wires, and
- ladders and step stools.

What is not known from this data is the condition of the equipment or the possibility that falls occurred due to characteristics inherent in the person (such as poor balance from a disease, or from a pre-existing visual impairment). It is conceivable that a ladder may have an un-sturdy handrail or that the steps were in poor repair leading to a fall.

Two of these environmental hazards as causative factors for falls are presented below: falls related to the steps, ladders, or stepping stools and falls occurring in the bathroom.

1. **Falls associated with steps, ladders, or stools**

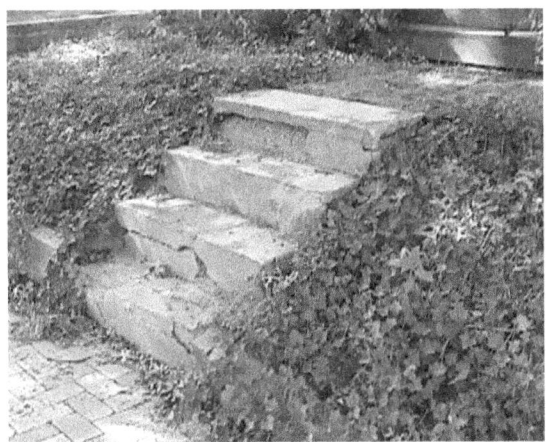

Figure 2-3 Poorly Maintained Steps

Falls from steps can occur from a variety of mechanisms ranging from the condition and height of the step to the sturdiness or presence of a hand-rail. The outdoor steps (see Figure 2-3) presented here possess all three problems related to condition, height, and lack of a hand-rail. Because of these steps are in very poor condition, they are apt to cause a fall when a person attempts to climb or descend them. The depth of the step poses additional problems for a person with lower extremity weakness, who might not be capable of lifting legs without the assistance of a hand-railing. The County Office on Aging can refer older persons to existing home repair "handyman" services for repair of steps or stairs in poor condition.

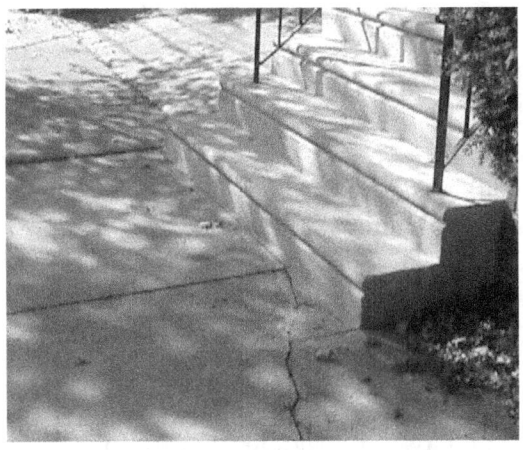

Figure 2-4 Hand rails on the second step

The other concern about steps relates to the hand-rail, especially when it is located on the second step as opposed to the first step (as seen in Figure 2-4). Hand-rails closest to the landing surface such as the first step or landing surface can guide the visually impaired person or add support when pre-existing conditions are present.

Ladder steps and steps on stepping stools are also potentially problematic due to the same underlying reasons - the condition of the step, the height of the step and the presence of sturdy hand-rails. Wobbly step stools may flip over.

2. Falls in the bathroom

The bathroom is a common place for falls. Bathtubs can be sites of accidental falls due to a slip. Accumulated soap film debris, use of oil-based emollients and other bathing solutions can contribute to slips and falls. Sometimes shiny tub surfaces may indicate such conditions are present. Missing or improperly placed grab bars/rails in or around the tub further contribute when the person is unable to steady himself or herself by holding on to a grab-bar. For these reasons, many persons choose to bathe sitting down or in a shower chair, use waterproof shoes with rubber soles providing an anti-slippage, or have tub mats that can help prevent a slip. Stores provide grab bars that can be clamped onto the tub edge providing assistance in and out of the tub. Some of these devices have adjustable heights.

3. Other hazardous areas

For certain age-groups such as young children and older adults, the home environment contains hazards that may increase the risk to fall. It is estimated that about one third of community dwelling older adults fall (NCIPC, 2007) [4] each year and falls among children are equally as high. Stair, crib and bed falls are common places for falls of younger people. Research on hazards in the home and risk of falls and injuries among older age groups has found that certain hazards increased the risk of falls in individuals compared to those people who had never fallen. [5] When hazardous toilet railings were present, the risk of recurrent falls significantly increased. Some specific hazards were associated with hip fracture: doormats, floor mats in traffic-ways, internal steps, seating, bed-lighting, bathtubs, bathmats and toileting. Overall, a person with a recent hip fracture was exposed to many more hazards - on average 6.3 - compared to those without a hip fracture. An analysis of multiple studies found that the most common factor associated with falls was an accident or environmental hazard. [6]

A home safety inspection can be professionally performed by a licensed occupational therapists or visiting nurse. Consumers can perform a room by room safety inspection, using the Home Safety Checklist, focusing on these high risk areas:

- Lighting
- Steps
- Doorways
- Floor surfaces
- Presence of obstacles like cords or throw rugs
- Bathrooms: tubs, showers and toilets – use of grab-bars and railings
- Seating
- Improper footwear

Improper footwear constitutes a hazard. A few studies have found evidence for risk of falls in older adults related to shoe-wear. In one study, greater heel height was associated with increased risk of a fall, whereas greater sole contact area was associated with reduced fall risk. [7] Shoes such as those worn by athletes appear to be beneficial for older adults to lower risks of falling. [8]

D. Environmental Falls in Healthcare Settings

In healthcare settings, *environmental falls* commonly occur from a spill or wet surface. [9, 10] Patients who do not wear non-skid or rubber soled slippers or shoes can experience a fall while ambulating across a linoleum floor. Beds, wheelchairs, and tables which do not have locked brakes can result in slips when the furniture rolls away from the patient.

Critical thinking question for the legal nurse consultant: Have you ever visited a nursing home or hospital and nearly slipped on the shiny floor surface on the unit? If you have, you should report it to the facility management. Chances are too, if you nearly fell, others might have also, or worse, actually fell and injured themselves. What types of surveillance or documentation are in place to verify that safety checks or environmental rounds are made so floors are safe to travel on, free of spills and slippery surfaces? The legal nurse consultant may suggest the attorney requests logs of safety checks performed by the housekeeping department. The attorney may also seek to determine if the facility used surveillance cameras and kept the recordings.

The environmental checklist performed in the healthcare setting includes all of the areas previously described in the home. However, the onus of responsibility for ensuring that the environments are safe emanates from Administration and rests upon all healthcare providers in the workforce - risk managers, housekeeping department, nursing and non-nursing personnel. Joint Commission recognizes the shared and collaborative work by all healthcare providers in its National Patient Safety Goals designed to maintain a safe healthcare environment. Typically, environmental rounds and safety checks are performed by discrete personnel or departments and are not uniformly shared by all departments.

Table 2-1 Examples of items to Examine on Environmental Safety Rounds

Items to check	Responses (Yes/No)	
Beds:		
Are beds in low rise locked positions?	Yes	No
Are locks in working order?	Yes	No
If the bed moves in locked position, replace/repair.	Yes	No
Are wheels of beds, equipment clean and free of debris?	Yes	No
If not, have wheels cleaned.		
Bed-side Stands/table tops:		
Are bed-side tables in locked positions?	Yes	No
Are locks in working order?	Yes	No
If bed-side table moves in locked position, replace/repair.	Yes	No
Chairs:		
Does chair have adjustable height?	Yes	No
Are locks used on wheels?	Yes	No
Canes/walkers:		
Are tips of canes in good repair?	Yes	No
Are walker tips in good repair?	Yes	No
If assistive device has torn tips, replace.		
Floor Surfaces:		
Are floor surfaces clear and free of spills?	Yes	No
Are floor surfaces slippery?	Yes	No
Is non-skid floor wax used?	Yes	No
Is the floor surface free of holes, cracks, or uneven areas?	Yes	No
Bathroom:		
Are grab-rails and hand-rails present and sturdy?	Yes	No
If not, repair or install.		
Does the call light work properly?	Yes	No
If not, repair.		
Is the toilet seat firmly affixed to the commode? If no, repair.	Yes	No
Room interior:		
Do call bells work?	Yes	No
Do cords easily disconnect from wall unit?	Yes	No
If yes, replace or repair.	Yes	No
Does the intercom system work?	Yes	No
Are lights in rooms working?	Yes	No
Is lighting bright and non-glare producing?	Yes	No
Are night-lights available?	Yes	No
Do night lights work?	Yes	No
Are grab-bars appropriate height and sturdy?	Yes	No
If not, replace or repair.		

Delegating environmental safety to all involved minimizes liability and potential errors of omissions when staff shortages occur. Use of an environmental safety checklist (see Table 2-1) facilitates a thorough inspection, pointing to areas that need corrective action.

E. Equipment Safety

Equipment safety depends on its proper functioning. This applies to devices and furniture. Equipment should be routinely checked for sturdiness and ability to perform properly. Side rails can be particularly hazardous if they are faulty or collapse when the patient leans on them for support. Specific protocols are recommended in Chapters 4 and 5 to address safety precautions in the healthcare setting.

Although a fall in a public place or in one's home or healthcare setting can occur solely due to an environmental hazard (and this is often assumed to be the case) a fall could also be related to alcohol or certain medications. These substances may cause drowsiness. Falls are correlated with pre-existing conditions resulting in loss of balance, lower extremity weakness, or a tendency for a lower limb to give out. Therefore, in the workplace where there is a high risk for fatal injury (such as falls off scaffolds), it is especially important that persons are educated about foreseeable and preventable events so that they can institute proactive measures to avoid personal injury.

F. Medications Related to Falls

Medications may be the underlying cause of the fall, as some drugs may suddenly lower heart rate or blood pressure. This condition is known as postural or orthostatic hypotension. Other potentially dangerous side effects include drowsiness, mental confusion, and problems with balance or loss of urinary control especially among older adults. All of these effects may lead to a slip and fall. [11-15] Persons may recognize an adverse effect, such as unsteadiness, loss of balance, or mental confusion that may lead to falls. Prompt notification of the physician/prescriber is needed to initiate corrective action. It is recommended that the nurse alert the prescriber for review of the need for the medication whenever a medication is suspected by the professional nurse as a contributor to a fall. Professional nurses who determine a medication is contraindicated are advised to consult a nursing supervisor. In these situations, the nurse may withhold the medication until it is reviewed by the prescriber. Pharmacological review of medications on a regular basis is another safeguard. Sometimes a medication can be substituted or doses lowered to manage symptoms associated with falling. Classifications of medications implicated in falls for older adults include psychotropic agents (benzodiazepines, sedatives/hypnotics, antidepressants, and neuroleptics), anti-arrhythmics, digoxin and diuretics. [16]

Critical thinking point for legal nurse consultants and nursing home clinicians: Examine the document which records the pharmacist's review of the medications prescribed to an elder. Determine if there were any recommendations to alter doses of any psychotropic medications. Were they followed by the prescriber? Is there any documentation of excessive sleepiness as a potential contributor to a fall?

G. Age-Related Changes Associated with Falling

There may be subtle changes in adults' organ systems as well as the presence of medical diseases (comorbidities) of an acute or chronic nature that contribute to falling. Experts agree that it is the comorbidity of aging related to changes and not age per se that increases the risk of falls. [17] Highlighted here are some of the visual and neuromuscular changes experienced by older adults.

1. Visual changes in the older adult include presbyopia - a reduction in accommodation. The effects of presbyopia are most obvious when descending the steps. Because of this condition, older adults may miss the last step (an important reason why the hand-rail must end on the landing surface).

2. Changes in the diameter of the pupil, a condition called "senile miosis", results in smaller pupils. Dimly lit rooms and hallways or surface edges that do not have bold contrasting colors can lead to trips and falls.
3. The presence of a cataract, more prevalent in older age groups and with certain conditions, obstructs central vision and can contribute to falls when steps or obstacles are not visualized. In a study of older adults with cataract, removal was associated with a reduced risk for recurrent falling. [18] Some older adults do not lift their feet high. If a reduced steppage height is evident, stumbles, trips and falls can occur when ascending steps or while walking on uneven surface. Also, transitioning from a flat floor surface to a thicker carpeted surface can produce similar falls. Neuromuscular changes include impaired ability to react to sudden loss of balance (from a push or trip) or impaired ability to maintain upright stance. [19]

H. Medical Causes of Falls

Medical causes such as seizure disorders or inner ear disturbances causing dizziness can be cited as contributors or antecedents to falling. These medical reasons vary among age-groups and can occur from acute or chronic diseases. [20-23] A common clinical example of a medically-related fall occurs when a person experiences lightheadedness when sitting or standing at the bedside. This symptom may correlate to a drop in blood pressure when standing. Patients prone to this problem need assistance with changing position, such as initially standing. Failure to assist patients who have a drop in blood pressure or complain of lightheadedness with transfer is negligent. However, a hospitalized patient or nursing home resident may stand up without calling for help. The question of the degree of supervision that should have been in place then arises. Patients who appear to have suffered a medically-caused fall should be further evaluated by the primary care provider or a specialist.

Table 2-2 Some Symptoms Associated with Falling by Older Adults

Dizziness
Lightheaded (spinning sensation such as vertigo)
Blacking out (loss of consciousness)
Loss of balance (sudden or chronic) "feeling wobbly"
Can't see (chronic or sudden loss of vision in one or both eyes)
Tiredness (chronic or sudden fatigue)
Sudden weakness in the legs or on one side of the body

Some common chronic diseases [such as arthritis of the lower extremities, or diabetes mellitus which in the end-stages can cause lower extremity loss of sensation (neuropathy)] can cause falling. In older years, the incidence of dementia (such as Alzheimer's disease) and neurological disorders like Parkinson's disease increases. These diseases impair judgment, affect walking and thinking, and frequently result in falling. Treatment of chronic diseases often includes medications, which may have adverse side effects associated or contributing to falls. Symptoms associated with diseases, medications, and other phenomena may be present at the time of the fall, prompting the practitioner to further investigate the cause of the symptom. For instance, dizziness or lightheadedness may be due to the new onset of a cardiac, circulatory, or inner ear disturbance. A review of some of the common symptoms associated with falling is presented in Table 2-2. [24]

I. Intrinsic Risk Factors Associated with Falls for an Older Adult

It is not always apparent why the fall occurred when a lawsuit is initiated because of a fall. A recent summary of 16 studies defined the most common risk factors for falls, listed here in the order of most frequent to least frequent:

- leg weakness,
- history of falls,
- gait deficit,
- balance deficit,
- use of an assistive device,
- visual deficit,
- arthritis,
- impaired ability to perform activities of daily living,
- depression,
- cognitive impairment, and
- age greater than 80.

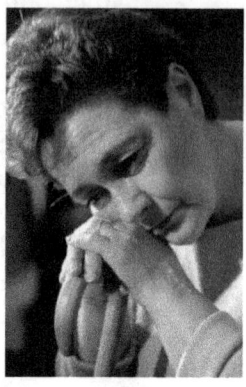

Figure 2-6: Use of an Assistive Device Increases Risk of Falls

Leg weakness increases the risk of falling by more than four times. The risk factors for *injurious* falls are the same factors for falls in general, with the addition of being female, the presence of at least two chronic conditions, and having a low body mass. [25, 26]

J. Risk Factor Assessment in the Medical Care Setting
The prevention of falls depends largely upon timely and accurate recognition and treatment (when possible) of the known causes of falls, as determined through one of two mechanisms:

- assessment of risk to fall (i.e., fall risk assessment)
- post-fall assessment (a comprehensive assessment of the person's fall history, circumstance and physical examination; see Chapter 3).

Generally, fall risk assessment is performed both in advance of a fall, as a screening measure (this is considered a primary level of prevention), and after a fall (this is considered a secondary level of prevention). Post-fall assessment is recognized as a secondary level of prevention. See Chapter 3 and 4 for further discussion of levels of prevention.

> The clinical review of cases takes into account many interactive dynamics related to the person who fell as well as the context or situation I which the fall occurred. Ideally, the medical record contains all of the necessary information needed to formulate an opinion on the cause of the fall with a reasonable degree of certainty. All factors are equally important in determining likely causes of falls.

Some of the areas reviewed to determine the cause of a fall include:

- the person's age at the time of the fall,
- a history of medical problems (chronic diseases and acute problems known from evidence-based medicine, which describe clinical practice based on the most valid and reliable research findings, to contribute or be the cause of the fall),
- current medications,
- functional status,

- mental status (delirium or level of consciousness),
- behavior (impulsivity, wandering or a history of getting lost),
- memory and recall,
- pertinent laboratory data such as electrolyte disturbances, low hemoglobin, blood sugar or oxygenation levels,
- vital signs (low blood pressure or orthostatic hypotension)
- gait and balance abilities related to turning or transferring, and
- any statements made by patients are often pertinent, such as descriptions of sudden symptoms such as dizziness when standing. These statements may be scattered throughout the chart or contained on the incident report form.

The patient's need for assistance or supervision is determined based on the history and physical examination and the plan of care. Interventions in place at the time of the fall may or may not be appropriate depending on the type of fall which is believed to have occurred. Review of the plan of care and interventions that were carried out is a key part of the clinical analysis of the fall.

This chapter has presented some of the common underlying reasons and risks to fall in various public and patient settings. In any setting, one fall is too many. Fall incidences are highest among older adults in institutional long-term care. The prevention of falls and fall-related injuries becomes the shared responsibility of all healthcare providers, professionals, administrators and staff. Chapter 3 addresses how falls can be prevented in these settings. Asking the right set of questions helps to determine why a fall may have occurred.

End Notes

[1] Davies, A. J., Steen, N., & Kenny, R. A. "Carotid sinus hypersensitivity is common in older patients presenting to an accident and emergency department with unexplained falls." *Age and Ageing,* 30(4), pgs. 273-274, 2001.

[2] Aging and Seniors. Available on the Internet at: http://www.phac-aspc.gc.ca/seniors-aines/pubs/seniors_falls/chapter3_e.htm

[3] Tinetti, M.E., et al. "Risk factors for serious injury during falls by older persons in the community", *Journal of the American Geriatrics Society* 43: pgs. 1214-21, 1995.

[4] National Center for Injury Prevention and Control (NCIPC) [Online]. Available on Internet at: http://www.cdc.gov/ncipc/ Accessed March 15, 2006.

[5] Clemson, L., Cumming, R.G., Roland, M "Case-control study of hazards in the home and risk of falls and hip fractures", Age and Ageing 25: pgs. 97-101, 1996.

[6] Komara, F. "The slippery slope: reducing fall risk in older adults", *Primary Care: Clinics in Office Practice, 32 (3), September 2005*

[7] Tencer, A.F., Koepsell, T.D., Wolf, M.E., Frankenfeld, C.L., Buchner, D.M., Kukull, W.A., LaCroix, A.Z., Larson, E.B., Tautvydas, M. "Biomechanical properties of shoes and risk of falls in older adults." Journal of the American Geriatrics Society 52:11, pgs. 1840-1846, 2004.

[8] Koepsell, T.D., Wolf, M.E., Buchner, D.M., Kukull, W.A., LaCroix, A.Z., & Tencer, A.F. et al (2004). "Footwear style and risk of falls in older adults". Journal of the American Geriatrics Society, 52 (9), 1495-1501

[9] Connell, B.R. "Role of the environment in falls prevention." *Clinics in Geriatric Medicine,* 12(4), pgs. 859-880, 1996.

[10] Gill, T. M., Williams, C. S., Robinson, J. T., & Tinetti, M. E. "A population based study of environmental hazards in the homes of older persons." *American Journal of Public Health,* 89(4), pgs. 553-556, 1999.

[11] Kelly, K. D., Pickett, W., Yiannakoulias, N., Rowe, B. H., Schopflocher, D. P., et al. "Medication use and falls in community-dwelling older persons." Age and Ageing, 32(5), pgs. 503-509, 2004.

[12] Smith, R. G. "Fall-contributing adverse effects of the most frequently prescribed drugs", *Journal of the American Podiatric Medical Association, 93(1), pgs. 42-50, 2003.*

[13] Ensrud, K.E., Blackwell, T.L., Mangione, C.M. Bowman, Whooley, Bauer, et al. "Study of Osteoporotic Fractures Research Group. Central nervous system-active medications and risk for falls in older women", Journal of the American Geriatrics Society, 50 (10); pgs. 1629-1637, 2002.

[14] Neutel, C. I. Perry, S., & Maxwell, C. "Medication use and risk of falls", *Pharmacoepidemiological Drug Safety, 11(2), pgs. 97-104, 2002.*

[15] Leipzig, R. M. Cumming, R. G., & Tinetti, M. E. "Drugs and falls in older people: A systematic review and meta-analysis II: Cardiac and analgesic drugs." Journal of the American Geriatrics Society, 47(1), pgs. 40-50, 1999.

[16] Id.

[17] See note 2.

[18] Brennan, S., Dewar, C., Sen, J., Clarke, D., Marshall, T., and Murray, P.I. "A prospective study of the rate of falls before and after cataract surgery", British Journal of Ophthalmology, 87: 560-562, 2003

[19] Maki, B.E., and W.E. McIllroy. "Effects of aging on control of stability", In L. Luxon et al. (eds), *A Textbook of Audiological Medicine. Clinical Aspects of Hearing and Balance.* London: Marin Dunitz Publishers, pp.671-90, 2003.

[20] Shaw, F. E. "Falls in cognitive impairment and dementia", *Clinical Geriatric Medicine,* 18(2), pgs.159-173, 2002.

[21] Stolze, H., Klebe, S., Zechlin, C., Baecker, C., Friege, L., & Deuschl, G. "Falls in frequent neurological diseases—prevalence, risk factors and etiology", Journal of Neurology, 251(1), pgs. 79-84, 2004.

[22] Ooi, W. L., Hossain, M., & Lipsitz, L. A. "The association between orthostatic hypotension and recurrent falls in nursing home residents", *American Journal of Medicine,* 108(2), pgs.106-111, 2000.

[23] Mukai, S., & Lipsitz, L. A. "Orthostatic hypotension", *Clinics in Geriatric Medicine,* 18(2), pgs. 253-268, 2002

[24] Gray-Miceli, D , Johnson, J.C, Strumpf, N.E. "A stepwise approach to a comprehensive post-fall assessment", Annals of Long-Term Care: Clinical Care and Aging 13 (12), pgs. 16-24, 2005

[25] See note 6.

[26] Rubenstein, L. and Josephson, K., "Falls and their prevention in elderly people: what does the evidence show?" Medical Clinics of North America, 90 (5) September 2006.

Prevention of Falls in the Hospital
by Deanna Gray-Miceli and Elizabeth Capezuti

CHAPTER 3

Chapter 3 Prevention of Falls in the Hospital
Deanna Gray-Miceli, DNSc, APRN, FAANP and Elizabeth Capezuti, PhD, RN, FAAN

A. General Issues Influencing Patient Safety and Quality Care

Healthcare professionals and organizational systems share responsibility to ensure the safety for patients in any medical care setting. The Institute of Medicine (IOM) acknowledges three domains of quality (care processes) toward this goal including:

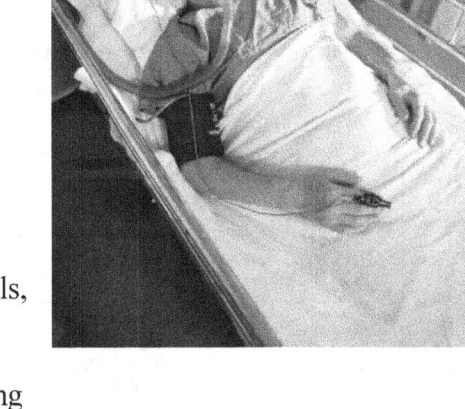

- safety (defined as freedom from accidental injury; ensuring patient safety involves the establishment of operational systems and processes that increase the reliability of patient care)
- practice consistent with current medical knowledge (such as best practices, incorporating evidenced-based medicine)
- customization (meeting consumer-specific values and expectations). [1]

Fall reduction activities are paramount for all individuals employed in a healthcare institution. This includes maintenance, housekeeping, volunteer services, any direct care providers such as nurses, nurses' aides, volunteers and primary health care professionals, to name a few. Professionals practicing in these institutions also ensure an added layer of safety by adhering to standards of practice and national recommendations for fall prevention. Practitioners caring for older adults may refer to several sources for recommendations to prevent falls and clinical practice guidelines on falls and fall risks. For general fall prevention care refer to:

- American Geriatrics Task Force on Fall Prevention [2] and
- Moreland's Guidelines for the Secondary Prevention of Falls. [3]

Professionals providing care to nursing home residents should refer to the prior recommendations and the clinical practice guidelines published by the American Medical Directors Association aimed at assisting practitioners to identify ways to modify risk factors and minimize the risk for injury due to falls. [4] This subject is covered in depth in Chapter 4. National professional recommendations for the prevention of falls and serious injury in children are available through the American Academy of Pediatrics Policy Statement on Falls from Heights, and the National SAFE KIDS Campaign initiatives that detail interventions for high risk activities which can result in injury. [5, 6, 7, 8]

Critical thinking point for legal nurse consultants: Determine what resources were used by a hospital to develop fall prevention policies and procedures. In some settings, the articles or books are listed in the policy or procedures. These references build the legal nurse consultant's library.

B. Levels of Prevention

The opportunities to prevent falls affect clinical practice for patients who have fallen or are at the greatest risk to fall. (See Figure 3-2.) *Primary prevention* refers to preventing the health-related event or disease. An example of primary prevention is screening for fall risk. In the public health arena, state departments of health produce brochures, educational programs and services, and also provide technical assistance to local departments of health for the general public of all ages. Advice focuses on fall prevention and safety in the home, on the playground, or in the work environment. Given the high incidence of serious and fatal falls in infants, toddlers and children as well as older adults, primary prevention through education and routine screening is essential.

Figure 3-2 Primary Prevention Interventions

Primary prevention interventions (children)
Wearing helmets when biking, using roller blades or skating
Using protective gear during athletic sports
Using bed-rails for toddlers
Avoiding baby walkers near steps; using safety gates
Utilizing window guards to avoid falls from windows

Primary prevention interventions (older adults)
Screening all older adults for fall history - over age 65
Participating in exercise programs for agility, strength, endurance and injury prevention
Using grab-rails in the tub/shower
Ensuring cane tips are not worn or frayed
Screening for risk for falling on admission (nursing home/medical care setting)
Screening for vision, gait and balance

Secondary prevention refers to early detection and intervention with the aim of reversing or retarding the progression of disease. Secondary prevention is aimed at preventing another fall. An assumption is that the first fall occurred by the same mechanism as the second fall. This *may* be true, but it does not necessarily *have* to be true. Consider a man who falls repeatedly for different reasons; first he slipped on a wet floor, then during the next fall, his arthritic knee buckled or his medication side-effect caused dizziness. Additional information on the secondary prevention of falls is available when caring for older adults. [9]

The Joint Commission requirements include the assessment and periodic reassessment of each patient's risk for falling, including the potential risks associated with the patient's medication regimen. Healthcare professionals are expected to take action to address identified risks through a fall reduction program. Fall assessment is a professional role and responsibility of nursing, medicine, pharmacy, and rehabilitation disciplines, as it lies within their scopes of practice. Typically, institutions will clearly identify in their policies and procedures the unique and combined roles of each discipline. Discipline-specific criteria are also referred to for guidelines and recommendations in professional practice. Considering the vast incidence of patient falls in medical care settings, team collaboration is essential.

Reduction of patient falls begins within a framework of team collaboration. Roles are shared, not solely prescribed. Characteristics of effective teams include:

- members monitor each other's performance, help each other; trust is essential
- giving and receiving feedback is a norm
- each person works to understand the other's role
- communication is real- senders check to ensure that messages are received as intended. [10]

In the process of creating a culture of safety, team members co-create a mutually reciprocal environment for patient safety that is rooted in open communication and accountability. Such a focus and change in organizational culture focuses on systems issues such as the need to strengthen safety practices.

Root cause analysis (RCA) has a place in identifying gaps and culprits leading to unsafe patient scenarios arising from sub-standard communication practices, policies and practices or management issues. These may include lack of training or knowledge by professionals (i.e., failure to maintain current practice) and failure to recognize the patient's values and wishes (individualizing care.)

C. Framework for Reducing Patient Falls (Adverse Events): Root Cause Analysis

1. Defining error

The Institute of Medicine (IOM) has defined error as the "failure of planned action to be completed as intended, the use of a wrong plan to achieve the aim." [11] Errors can occur related to problems in practice, products, procedures or systems. The IOM notes that not all errors end in injury. A culture of safety assumes that mistakes are unintentional and a wide variety of errors can occur. In adverse event reporting, a continuous process of evaluation and re-evaluation ensures that errors (sentinel events) or potential errors (near misses) are systematically identified and eliminated from reoccurring. RCA is a retrospective approach to error analysis. [12] RCA is used in medicine and nursing for the investigation of sentinel events, and in 1997 was mandated by the Joint Commission for use in the investigation of sentinel events in accredited hospitals. [13] RCA has several methodological limitations as it represents an uncontrolled case study. The occurrence of accidents is highly unpredictable; it is impossible to know if the root cause established by the analysis is the cause of the accident. [14] Table 3-1 describes the minimum scope of RCA for fall-related sentinel events.

Table 3-1 Root Cause Analysis Matrix: Minimum Scope of Root Cause Analysis for Specific types of Sentinel Events: Fall Related. Modified from TJC, October 2005, Root Cause Analysis Matrix

Items to Include in Analysis	Comments related to fall prevention
Physical assessment process	Was a fall history and physical completed?
Patient observation process	Were there changes in level of consciousness or level of function? Was there a post-fall injury?
Care planning process	Was a care plan identified for fall risks? Did the plan of care address the individual causes of this patient's fall?
Continuum of care	Is there ongoing evaluation and monitoring of the patient by multiple disciplines such as medicine, physical therapy as well as nursing?
Staffing levels	Does the facility provide adequate staffing to attend to patients at highest risk for serious injury or frequent falling?
Orientation and training of staff	Does the facility provide detailed fall-focused educational inservices about risks for falling, causes of falls and appropriate interventions?
Competency assessment/training	Is staff evaluated by nursing administration

Items to Include in Analysis	Comments related to fall prevention
	for their capabilities of performing necessary elements of a post fall assessment such as neurological checks or checking patients for orthostatic hypotension?
Communication with patients and families	Does the patient have an understanding of the medical evaluation for a fall? Is the family aware of the patient's history of recurrent falling?
Communication with staff members	Are there appropriate and adequate systems of communication utilized by a facility so that all staff are aware of the need to identify risks for falls, importance of fall reporting, and monitoring patients post-fall?
Availability of information	When patients cannot communicate adequately or reliability about their falls, what sources of information do facility and staff rely on? Is this documented in the fall policy and procedure?
Equipment maintenance management	Equipment includes furnishings- hardware, bar, hooks, rods, preventing and fixing ripples in rugs, broken steps, and dim lighting. Is there regular inspection and repair of such items?
Medication management	Are medications that increase risk to fall regularly reviewed by the pharmacist, prescriber, nurse and team?

2. Process and components of root cause analysis

According to Reason's 1991 multi-causal theory "Swiss Cheese" diagram, there are many organizational triggers leading to adverse events. These triggers include:

- lack of procedures
- punitive policies
- production pressures
- mixed messages
- zero fault tolerance
- sporadic training
- attention distractions
- deferred maintenance
- clumsy technology

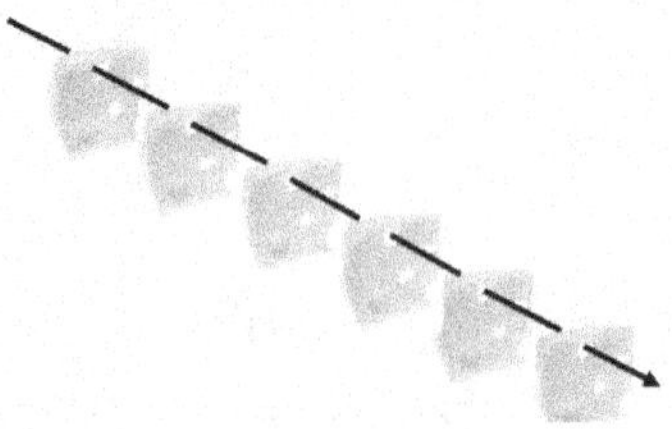

Figure 3-3 Swiss cheese model. The holes in the Swiss cheese line up to permit an injury to occur.

Solutions to these triggers are directed within policies and procedures, professional teams, individual professions, environmental safety and equipment (as outlined by Joint Commission). By using a checklist based on a framework for a RCA, an action plan can be created in response to a sentinel event. Table 3-2 includes a sample of questions included in such a framework which is completed by organizations to evaluate the cause of the sentinel event so that corrective action can take place. Included are the level of analysis, key questions, findings, identification of root cause, asking why and action taken. Hospitals are required to complete a RCA for each sentinel event and in certain states report these findings to the state department of health, which monitors such events.

Table 3-2 Sample Questions for a Root Cause Analysis in Response to a Sentinel Event. Adapted from TJC, October, 2005, Root Cause Analysis Matrix.

Level of analysis	Questions
1. What happened?	What are the details? When did the event occur? What area or service was impacted?
2. Why did it happen?	What are the steps in the process?
3. What were the most proximate factors?	What human factors were relevant to the outcome? How did the equipment performance affect the outcome? What factors directly affected the outcome? Are they truly beyond the organization's control? Are there any other factors that have directly influenced this outcome? What other areas or services are impacted?
4. Why did that happen?	To what degree is staff properly qualified and currently competent for their responsibilities?

D. Measures to Prevent Patient Falls

1. Communication

Joint Commission has found after performing an analysis of root causes of sentinel events, that poor communication accounted for the major underlying reason for many of the adverse events reported.[15] Consider this case tried for poor or inadequate communication:

> In *Conrad v. Carondelet Health Network d/b/a St. Mary's Hospital*, the plaintiff was a surgery patient at the defendant hospital. She claimed although she rang for a nurse numerous times after midnight, no one came to her assistance. When she proceeded to the restroom on her own, she fell and sustained a dislocated fracture of the shoulder. The plaintiff claimed that the defendant failed to provide adequate staff supervision. The verdict was for the defense.[16]

Errors in communication can be addressed through improved systems of monitoring or calling for assistance and through improved documentation tools. Nursing personnel in medical care facilities must become better equipped to respond to patient needs in a timely and accurate fashion. Some simple solutions include the use of video surveillance in non-private areas, intercom systems, frequent observation, use of unlicensed assistive personnel to perform additional rounds of observation, and one on one assistance where indicated for patients who may be confused or delirious and demonstrate unpredictable behavior because of poor impulse control or loss of memory.

2. Documentation

Proper documentation is a written form of good communication about patient problems such as falls. Research has found multiple and duplicative information charted about patient falls. [17] Centralized, streamlined versions are essential for staff compliance, ideally limited to a few non-duplicative sources. Documentation about falls must also be comprehensive and lead the practitioner and team to a determination of a comprehensive plan of care. Problem-oriented medical records should identify fall risk or fall history and the presence of injury outcomes. Interdisciplinary plans of care also address fall prevention through individualized plans of care.

There should be documentation on the post-fall assessment or in the incident report and/or nurses' note, progress note or post-fall assessment tool describing:

- specific circumstances preceding the fall (including associated symptoms such as lightheadedness, weakness, or palpitations as well as medications administered and environmental conditions such as lighting and floor surface),
- results of the immediate physical examination (including vital signs, musculoskeletal, neurologic, cardiovascular, and functional assessment),
- treatment(s) administered, and
- phone calls to the staff member's supervisor, and the patient's attending physician and emergency contact.

Hospital reports containing this information, such as incident reports, are routinely reviewed by the medical director and nurse administrator and signed (see Figure 3-4 for more detail).

Figure 3-4 Comprehensive Post Fall Note

3/12/07 5:00 AM: Ms. S., a 86-year-old woman was getting up from bed to walk to the bathroom and suddenly felt dizzy. Recalls falling to the ground about 4:30 am. Review of systems reveals dizziness for about 2 days, poor vision, and now has a headache and urinary frequency x 2 days. Denies loss of consciousness, focal weakness, slurred speech or chest pain. PMH includes hypertension, TIA and arthritis of the knees. Medications - unchanged. Uses a walker for distance. Vitals: 98.6-88-20 BP supine 140/70 and 122/60 standing. Awake and alert, no focal neurological or muscular deficits. Gait steady with walker. Apical 88 and regular. Lungs clear. No focal injury. Fall risk assessment performed: deficits in vision, presence of orthostatic hypotension. Assisted back to bed, call bell in place. Patient reassured. Family and physician notified. Will institute fall precautions, post-fall protocol and review incident with team and primary physician. In the interim will use bedpan at night if needed. See plan of care for more details. Ms. XXX RN.

A hospital which utilizes a coordinated team approach to fall monitoring will analyze individual case occurrences of falls as well as unit-based fall incidences, continually re-evaluating and determining appropriate plans of care.

More information related to documentation is contained in Appendix Two.

> ***Critical thinking point for the legal nurse consultant:*** How does the legal nurse consultant know if a patient actually fell in a medical care setting?

There are several mechanisms for verifying if a fall and associated injury occurred. Video surveillance may be available for review and analysis in a public setting within a medical care setting such as a waiting room or entrance to the facility. Performing a historical "look back" when reviewing old records can help to establish if any particular patterns emerge whereby an injury may be alleged, but never occurred. Another mechanism is to analyze the injury type and trajectory of impact. Consider if an injury could occur according to the description provided by the falling person. From a clinical stance, knowing if the person is receiving a blood thinner medication or has a bleeding disorder can help explain the severity of the injury and its duration. Knowledge of the standard rate of change in skin discoloration following an injury can help pinpoint the time of occurrence.

- Blue, purple or black colors may occur from one hour of bruising until resolution.
- Red has no bearing on the age of the bruise because it may occur at any time.
- A bruise with yellow must be older than 18 hours. [18]

Healthcare providers may become suspicious when the injuries do not match the explanation of how they occurred. Although this disparity may be encountered anywhere in healthcare, it is most evident in physician offices and emergency departments. Child abuse may be suspected.

> ***Critical thinking point for clinicians***: A mother brings her child to the emergency department. The child has fading yellow bruises on her face and neck. No other bruises are seen. Mom says, "She fell down the stairs an hour ago."

The reasons the question of child abuse should be raised include:

- The color of bruise is not consistent with time frame of injury.
- Additional bruises or abrasions would be expected if a fall of this nature occurred.
- The face is the most common site of bruising when a child is abused.

At times, the way the fall occurred is not accurately reported. Nurses, nursing aides, and others may panic after the fall and fail to either report the fall, or provide inaccurate information about how the fall occurred. This attempted cover up often backfires when others become suspicious based on additional assessment data. Case One and Case Two in Appendix Two show examples of such cases.

3. Environmental and equipment safety

A culture of safety assumes that all patient-related equipment is not only properly checked for adequate functioning regularly, but that all equipment that patients encounter is safe. Many procedures performed in the hospital setting are associated with risks. All members of the hospital staff are responsible for ensuring that issues of patient safety are identified and adhered to. Consider these cases:

In *Robert Anthony v. Riddle Memorial Hospital*, the 90-year-old plaintiff became agitated and was sedated at the emergency department. After he was admitted to the hospital in an unresponsive and sedated state, ten hours later he was found on the floor, having fallen from bed. He suffered a fractured femur, which required two surgeries to repair. The plaintiff claimed the defendant failed to apply proper fall precautions, including keeping bed rails in the up position and establishing a toilet schedule. According to the plaintiff, his diagnosis established him as a fall risk. The defendant denied any negligence. A $200,000 verdict was returned with a finding of 25 percent fault on the part of the plaintiff. The verdict was molded to $150,000. [19]

Refer to Chapter 5 for a discussion on the role of side rails, if any, in preventing falls.

In *Neve v. Sunrise Hospital and Medical Center*, a 55-year-old plaintiff was admitted to the hospital with symptoms and a history of breathing difficulty, pulmonary edema, high blood pressure, and chronic obstructive pulmonary disease. She collapsed during transfer from her hospital bed to an MRI table and struck her head. The plaintiff claimed that she experienced orthostatic hypotension as a result of medication, low blood pressure, and her bedridden state when she attempted to move. The plaintiff claimed the defendant failed to provide adequate personnel. The jury awarded $200,000. [20]

4. Fall risk assessment
a. General issues related to measures of fall risk

There are many fall risk assessment tools available for use with older adults in either acute care hospitals or in nursing homes. These risk assessments are used as screening tools for the primary prevention of falls when identified risks are modified or in the secondary prevention of patient falls. Their scope and empirical testing (in term of validity, reliability, and prediction) vary, but should be ascertained prior to use to ensure that they gather both valid and reliable information.

> Current Joint Commission standards and professional recommendations from national organizations (American Geriatric Society and the American Medical Directors Association) recommend use of fall risk assessments with patients either at risk or who have fallen.

Perell's review of the 1984 to 2001 literature identified 20 fall risk tools, 15 of which were nursing assessment tools. Of these, 12 were used in for inpatient settings and 3 were designated for nursing home use. [21] Some of the risk assessment tools were the Morse Fall Scale, Heindrich Fall Risk Model, Fall Prediction Index, Stratify, Assessment for High Risk to Fall and High Risk for Falls Assessment. Most of these tools identified co-morbid patient characteristics and conditions associated with falling such as:

- alteration in mental status or cognitive impairment,
- history of a fall,
- mobility impairment due to gait or balance problems or both,
- secondary or specific diagnosis known to affect fall risk (such as orthostatic hypotension or urinary incontinence),
- certain medications or polypharmacy,
- sensory deficits (such as visual deficits), and
- age.

Most of the tools reviewed by Perell [22] for use in in-patient settings have cut-off scores, sensitivity, specificity, and other information needed to determine predictive validity. Validity was not reported for the three risk assessment tools for use in nursing homes.

Fall risk tools commonly used by professional and available in the public domain typically include:

- level of consciousness or cognition,
- history of previous fall,
- systolic blood pressure,
- ambulation status,
- visual status,
- gait and balance,
- predisposing diseases and medications. (See Table 3-3).

These tools reflect both static characteristics (such as past medical history) and dynamic interactions (such as current orthostatic blood pressure or level of consciousness). Furthermore, these tools are administered prior to a fall, as well as during a post-fall assessment. They do not address the underlying causes of an actual fall, the primary purpose of the post-fall assessment.

> Fall risk assessment is based on identifying the contributions of several risk factors for falls. Prudent medical and nursing care is directed towards identifying and modifying- in advance- the risks for falls. Revision of the plan of care is based on the recognition of the need to make changes to lessen the risk of subsequent falls.

Currently, there are no pediatric fall risk assessment tools in the public domain. Hospitals for children have referred to medical management organizations for available benchmarks.[23] In some cases, such hospitals have developed their own instruments for assessment based on the criteria included for older adults. As mentioned previously, factors covered in the risk assessment also occur in younger ages as risks to fall or causes to fall.

Table 3-3 Some Components of Fall Risk Assessments

Parameter	Status/condition
Level of consciousness/mental status	Alert, disoriented, confused
History of falls (past 3 months)	No falls (1-4 or more)
Ambulation status	Ambulatory, chair bound, bed bound
Vision Status	Adequate, poor, blind
Gait/balance	Gait and balance normal Change in gait pattern with walking Jerking or unstable when turning Requires use of assistive device
Systolic Blood Pressure	No drop noted, drops more than 20mm Hg

It is the primary responsibility of the healthcare team (physician, nurse and physical therapist) to evaluate a patient's risk for falling. As part of this assessment, the pharmacist is responsible to regularly assess known medication effects.

E. Fall Risk Assessment versus Post-fall Assessment

Fall risk assessment and post fall assessment are two inter-related but distinct components of fall prevention. The importance of both is recognized by professional societies and national organizations. These two approaches are complimentary and in the case of post-fall assessment for older adults, fall risk assessment alone does not provide the necessary items required to perform a comprehensive post fall assessment.

Current Joint Commission standards and professional recommendations from national organizations (American Geriatric Society and the American Medical Directors Association) recommend a thorough post-fall evaluation for older patients who have fallen.

1. Post-fall assessment

The post-fall assessment or evaluation takes into account consideration of the many inter-related factors, diseases, and medications that predispose patients to falling. A post-fall assessment is comprehensive enough to answer the question of why a fall occurred. (See Figure 3-5.) Typically reviewed are past medical problems, medications used, current or on-going medical problems, functional assessment, a physical examination, and evaluation of the presence or absence of cognitive disorders such as dementia or Parkinson's disease. A comprehensive post-fall assessment is performed routinely by geriatric fall experts which include persons trained in geriatrics or advanced practice gerontological nursing. Elements of the post-fall assessment can be designated to nursing personnel.

Figure 3-6 lists items typically included in a post-fall assessment and performed by geriatric specialists in falls. In the absence of the availability of such a trained specialist, post-fall assessments such as this can be conducted by professional registered nurses or nurse generalists with the proper post-fall assessment documentation tools, and with training. Current post-fall assessment tools lack sufficient content to determine why a fall occurred. In previous research, the author found that their content did not reflect national recommendations for fall prevention. [24] Because of the lack of a uniform post-fall assessment tool, a post-fall assessment tool was developed and validated for use by registered nurses in nursing home facilities by the author. [25, 26] See Figure 3-7, located at the end of the chapter, for an outline of essential domains comprising this tool. This type of post-fall assessment provides more comprehensive information about potential etiology than fall risk assessment alone does, although both have an important place in the assessment of the falling person. One does not replace the other, rather they are complementary.

Figure 3-5 Questions to Ask to Determine What Happened Before, During, and After a Fall

History of the Fall
Describe your recent fall, and everything you recall. What did you experience?
What were you doing at the time of the fall - walking, moving, running, going to sit down, and so on?
Were you alone or was there someone present or nearby? Did you get up independently or have to call for help?
What happened when you got up?
Did you report your fall to your physician or nurse?
Did you seek medical attention in the hospital or emergency room or physician office?
What were you told, if anything, about why you fell?
Were any studies ordered or were you given any instruction on what to do?

Immediately following a fall, it is standard of care for the RN to perform an assessment to determine the nature and extent of any injury and the status of the patient. Circumstantial information is documented like the location, time, presence of witnesses, patient's statements and vital signs. This information is of limited usefulness in determining why the fall occurred. Thus, facilities and staff are better prepared to deal with the issue of falling when a more comprehensive approach is utilized that incorporates focused histories, situational contexts, issue of environment, equipment and devices as well as outcomes of the fall. Typically, registered nurse staff use nursing assessment forms to accomplish this as well as re-evaluate fall risk. At some future point (this may vary from that day to up to one week later), registered nurses discuss this information with the interdisciplinary team and revise, as needed, the plan of care.

Critical thinking point for legal nurse consultants: The clinical review of fall cases takes into account many interactive dynamics related to the person who fell as well as the context or situation in which the fall occurred. Ideally, the medical record contains all of the necessary information needed to assimilate an opinion with a reasonable degree of certainty. All factors are equally important in determining likely risks and causes.

Some of the areas recommended for review by the American Geriatrics Society Guidelines for Fall Prevention in the Elderly comprising the core components of a comprehensive post-fall assessment are included below. Note that geriatric specialists such as advance practice nurses or physicians typically perform these elements, but that most items can be elicited by the registered nurse.

Figure 3-6 Components of a Post Fall Assessment Tool

1. History of the Falling Event & Past Medical History
   - Age of the person
   - Statements made by the person about the fall, what he or she was doing or feeling such as sudden events like dizziness with standing. These statements may be scattered throughout the chart or contained on the incident report form.
   - Review of systems- review of pertinent symptoms such as headache or leg weakness
   - Review of medical problems (searching for chronic diseases and acute problems known from evidence-based medicine to contribute or be the cause of the fall), review of fall risk assessment factors
   - Current medications
   - Current functional status including basic activities of daily living, impulsivity, wandering or a history of getting lost
2. Physical examination
   - Vital signs including orthostatic blood pressures
   - Vision
   - Neurological assessment including mental status in terms of level of
   - consciousness, presence of focal, new deficits, gait and balance assessment,
   - muscular strength, memory and recall
   - Presence of physical injury
3. Review of pertinent laboratory data such as electrolyte disturbances, blood counts, oxygenation levels

The need for assistance or supervision is determined based on findings from the history and physical examination inclusive of a review of risks. Interventions are developed in the plan of care to address risks and associated causes. Review of the plan of care and interventions that were carried out is a key part of the clinical analysis of the fall.

The standard of care calls for assessment and re-evaluation of the patient's condition following a fall. This will be accomplished in an immediate post-fall period and should continue in the interim post fall period which may last for several days or even weeks.

2. Post-fall treatment

A patient should never be moved or transferred immediately after a fall until it is ascertained that the person has not suffered a head injury or spinal fracture. Injury may be worsened by movement without appropriate equipment such as a spinal immobilization board. A nurse, preferably a registered nurse, should touch the patient's joints and back to detect any deformities suggestive of a fracture or dislocation. If none are found, then the nurse should move each joint to reveal any limitations of movement, possibly indicating a fracture or sprain. Vital signs (pulse, blood pressure, and respiratory rate) are taken to detect signs of shock, heart dysrhythmia, or lung disorder secondary to rib fracture. A change in mental status is noted since it may suggest head trauma or shock. Any complaints of pain after a fall should be treated as if there was a fracture. The appropriate x-rays should be taken.

If a fracture or head trauma is suspected, the patient should be immediately evaluated by a physician, nurse practitioner, or physician assistant to rule out serious, life-threatening injuries. If the suspected injury occurs when a physician, nurse practitioner, or physician assistant is not readily available and will not be accessible for several hours, the patient should be transferred to the nearest hospital's emergency department. Failure to do so may lead to complications or death.

In *Anonymous Eighty-Seven Year-Old Male v. Defendant Nursing Home*, an 87-year-old man had been a resident of the defendant nursing home since 1996. He began falling in late 1999. During the year 2000, there was documentation of more than fifteen falls. In January 2001, the nursing home staff was found to have failed to use fall-prevention devices. In February 2001, the facility staff again failed to use the safety devices. As a result of that failure, the resident fell and sustained bilateral fractured hips. The resident was not transferred to a hospital for assessment and surgery repair for seven days after the fall. Action against the nursing facility was settled for $450,000. [27]

F. General Issues to Consider Regarding Patient Falling

1. Autonomy

Quality care for any patient requires primary practitioners to engage in dialogue about care rendered or planned that is respectful of patient values, beliefs and wishes. An integral component of communication and subsequent intervention entails risk sharing and negotiating acceptance of risk. Practitioners begin by choosing the least restrictive intervention that allows for maximum autonomy, independence, and individuality while also ensuring safety. Incidences do occur however, when it is not medically advisable or prudent care for a patient to perform an activity without assistance. Cognitively intact and medically stable patients who disregard nursing or medical instructions and get up unassisted may be at risk to fall. The standard of care requires that prior discussion and communication of this potential risk is stressed with patients or family caregivers. The geriatric literature further reports older adults' risk-taking behavior and situations which might predispose them to injury. In a medical care setting, practitioners and patients share in a responsibility to balance safety, fall prevention, independence, and respect for autonomy.

2. Medical stability

In some situations, older adult patients are incapable of making complex decisions because of diseases or syndromes such as Alzheimer's disease or delirium, to name a few. Individuals may be medically unstable but capable of making complex decisions; primary practitioners must act on their behalf to ensure safety by following professional codes of ethics and fundamental ethical principles, such as "do no harm". A case example is used to illustrate the interface between patient safety, medical stability, and autonomous decision-making among older adults who have fallen or are at high risk to fall again.

> In an acute care hospital, a 71-year-old, otherwise healthy female (cognitively intact, possessing decision-capacity with no prior fall history) was preparing for discharge home following a four day stay for routine appendectomy. Feeling well the day prior to her discharge, she insisted on getting up out of bed and taking a shower in the bathroom. The primary care nurse agreed, despite knowledge that the patient had a 102° temperature that morning and laboratory data showed a white-blood count greater than 30,000 indicative of an infection. During transit to the bathroom accompanied by the nurse, the patient complained of feeling suddenly "weak and very dizzy". The nurse sat the patient down in a chair, and left to get a blood pressure cuff. Upon returning, she found the patient lying in a pool of blood, dazed and unconscious.

> In this situation, an appropriate standard of care was not followed by the nurse in caring for this patient with an infection and a change in her medical stability from stable to unstable. Shared decision-making about risks and alternative actions did not take place. Alternative action could have been implemented by setting the patient up with a basin for a bed bath.

G. Hospital Policies and Procedures for Fall Reduction

Given the previous situation, communication and shared decision making are integral components of any fall prevention intervention. It is an appropriate standard of care to discuss this with older adults to learn of their wishes for future care planning, and to document such discussions. Team meetings can help to facilitate this dialogue.

In any hospital, policies for patient care related to fall screening (primary prevention), fall detection, reporting, documentation, and fall monitoring should be in place. The policy begins with defining a fall. Fall risk screening tools should be validated and empirically tested and not simply contrived by staff to fill a void. There are many fall risk tools appropriate for either general hospitals or nursing home settings in the public domain and available for purchase. The tools should be referred to by name, such as the Heinrich II tool or the Morse Scale. Their purposes, administration, and results are typically described and sample copies presented in the policy and procedure manual.

Critical thinking point for clinicians: Does your facility have a standardized fall risk assessment? How often should it be completed? Does the policy direct staff to complete the risk assessment when the condition of the patient changes? Are levels of risk well defined? Does staff know how to use the form? Has auditing been completed to determine if the form or risk assessment is being correctly used?

Methods for intercepting falls should be clear. For instance, are staff relying on alarms that sound for detection of a fall, or is staff required to routinely observe patients? Rounds can be assigned to a designated staff member to walk around the unit and check on the status of residents. Other types of clinical rounds occur when the registered nurse staff walks around the unit with the on-coming shift to give report as opposed to listening to a tape-recorded report or verbal report.

The channels for communication of fall reporting need to be clear. Falls are typically reported to the charge nurse by staff members or the patients themselves and then communicated to other team members via the nursing plan of care. Each patient should have an individualized plan of care directed at the potential cause of the fall, whenever known.

Table 3-4 presents a plan of care for an older adult with known risks for falling [poor vision, recent evidence of orthostatic hypotension and getting up at night to urinate; as described in Figure 3-4]. Note that the selected interventions always depend on the medical stability of the patient as determined by the nursing assessment and subsequent judgment as well as the physician or primary care provider's orders. Ideally, a fall plan of care such as this refers the registered nurse to appropriate protocol for further assessment and management. In the instance of neurological checks post-fall, separate protocols specify the frequency, length of time and progression of neurological checks. Neurological checks may be done every shift, every 4 hours or even every 15 minutes when nurses care for medically stable patients post-fall. It all depends on the stability of the patient and the nursing/medical judgment at that time. Neurological checks may be ordered more frequently to detect acute head injury post-fall after patients have unwitnessed falls, or for those who report new symptoms of headache or other pertinent neurological symptoms.

Frequently falling patients should be monitored; each fall should be designated by a number so that the frequency does not get lost in the medical record. Falls are documented internally by use of incident report forms. These forms are limited in information. In many parts of the United States, they are discoverable during litigation and thus often contain minimal information. They typically describe what happened and contain mostly circumstantial information about the fall. In all instances, patients (children and adults) should receive a comprehensive post-fall assessment performed by the registered nurse and then conveyed to the primary practitioner, which is designed to answer why the fall occurred. In addition, fall risk is reassessed looking for correctable situations.

Table 3-4 Care Plan for Addressing Risk for Falls

Goals	Interventions	Evaluation
1. Prevent falls due to: a) Poor vision	1a. Refer to ophthalmologist, perform environmental safety check, assist with ADLs as needed, use corrective lens	1a. Cataract removal scheduled
b) New orthostatic hypotension (OH)	1b. Check orthostatic BPs every shift x 3 days and report findings to physician provider; instruct patient to dangle, use TED stockings, refer to primary provider for work-up	1b. OH managed with TED stockings
c) Nocturnal urinary frequency	1c. Evaluate cause of urinary frequency while also providing patient with assistance at night; perform frequent toileting rounds	1c. Urinary frequency stopped once urinary infection treated
2. Rule-out post fall head trauma	2. Neurological checks every 15 min x 2 hours; then follow protocol; assess headache regularly, report increase immediately or if headache unrelieved with analgesia to primary provider; discuss with physician need for additional tests such as a head CAT Scan; place on frequent observation (walking rounds); consider 1:1 observations.	2. Headache persists. CAT scan ordered, neurological consult to be done

H. Prevention of Falls in the Institutionalized Patient

Fall and injury risk is often due to several factors, thus, the best intervention strategy for older adults is multifactorial and individualized to each patient's particular risk factors. [28, 29, 30] Two important systematic reviews of over one hundred combined clinical trials also concluded that multifactorial, multidisciplinary falls risk assessments and management are the most effective interventions. [31, 32]

Addressing individual risk factors is crucial in a falls management program. For example, patients with dementia and cognitive impairment fall more often than their counterparts and deserve close attention in prevention efforts. [33] In addition to addressing individual risk factors, facility-wide prevention strategies are also an important component of reducing fall risk. For example, colored vests or color-coded stickers to identify those at high risk for falls may be placed on the patient's wrist identification, wheelchair, room entrance, and bed. This intervention heightens awareness of the patient's risk to fall or to elope from the facility. Education of staff regarding risk factors and interventions is the cornerstone of any fall reduction efforts. Staff education and development of individual care plans for fall prevention may be facilitated by a nursing or rehabilitation consultant or a multidisciplinary falls consultation team. [34] Fall consultation services with structured, comprehensive, individualized assessment and safety recommendations have been shown to significantly reduce falls in the nursing home by 19 percent and injurious falls by 31 percent. [35] Not only do such programs have beneficial resident outcomes, but they are also cost-effective.

A falls reduction committee can also play an important role in fall prevention. A committee that brings together clinical staff (nursing, medicine, rehabilitation, and social work) with those responsible for maintaining a safe environment (administration, maintenance, and housekeeping) will result in clinically useful environmental modifications to prevent falls and injuries for both patients and staff. The committee should regularly review fall and injury statistics as well as analyze incident reports for patterns or trends that may lead to new fall prevention strategies. The goals of a falls reduction committee is best achieved within a Continuous Quality Improvement or Quality Assurance model. [36] The minutes of these meetings should demonstrate the facility's commitment to implementing changes geared toward fall prevention. The facility's policy and procedure manual will also define the facility's approach to fall prevention.

1. Prevention of falls in the hospitalized elderly [37]

There is evidence that falls in hospitals can be reduced, [38, 39] therefore, it is important to identify high risk patients so that specialized interventions can be implemented. All patients should be assessed for risk for falling at the time of hospital admission, and upon transfer to a different patient care unit. The initial fall risk assessment is usually part of the nursing admission history that is completed by the registered nurse who admits the patient. Patients are periodically reassessed for fall risk (per shift, daily, or weekly) depending on the acuity of the patient and hospital policy. A falls risk assessment can determine objectively whether a patient is at risk for falls. [40] Based on the assessment, staff can then develop a care plan that addresses fall prevention for the patient at risk. This may include referral to physical or occupational therapy for further risk assessment of areas identified like gait or balance impairment, and review of identified risks associated with changes in mental status or medications. Specific scores on the risk assessment trigger either further assessment or nursing interventions, which can range from simple interventions such as placing the call bell within reach of the patient to more technological interventions such as the use of bed exit alarms or mobility alarms.

When a patient falls while hospitalized, the immediate action taken by the registered nurse or the healthcare professional who finds the patient is to assess for physical injury. After this assessment, the registered nurse contacts the patient's primary care provider to report the incident. An occurrence report is completed, which documents the circumstances of the fall, and is forwarded to risk management. In some institutions, there has been a move to a more involved post-fall assessment. This assessment is completed by the registered nurse caring for the patient, but may, in some institutions, be completed by a geriatric advanced practice nurse who specializes in falls. The goal of the post-fall assessment is to look further and see what other causative factors may be involved. Post-fall assessments are not universally present in the acute care setting, and when in place, vary greatly in the amount and type of information they collect.

The patient is reassessed post-fall using the fall risk assessment tool. In many of the tools, the fall places the patient at a different risk level and other interventions are implemented. If a patient has been determined to be at risk of falling, or has fallen, then a thorough evaluation of amenable risk factors contributing to future risk should be conducted. Interventions to reduce the risk for falls need to be targeted to the individual and his/her specific risk factors. [41] Interventions that are related to extrinsic factors include removing clutter from the patient's room and hallway, ensuring that the bed is at a safe height, providing proper footwear, and placing non-skid strips on the floor and in the bathroom. [42]

Interventions targeted at intrinsic risk factors including a thorough review of medications to evaluate their potential for increasing fall risk is warranted and as well as looking at the necessity of medications. Avoiding the use of psychotropic medications as well as overall limiting the number of medications administered are important considerations. Bed alarms, monitors, and devices to alert staff when patients attempt to move without assistance are often useful in cognitively impaired patients. [43] Many falls are related to toileting, so interventions to make this safer are important. Offering commodes and scheduled toileting is useful in eliminating unsupervised trips to the bathroom. Ensuring that the bathroom is safe, with the use of raised toilet seats and grab bars, is indicated.[44]

All healthcare providers and professionals share in developing and evaluating plans of care for ensuring patient safety in the hospital consistent with the creation of an interdisciplinary culture of safety.

---

2. Prevention of falls in hospitalized children

The Joint Commission requirements for fall risk assessment and fall prevention are not age-specific. Hospitalized children fall, thus mandating the development of risk assessment and post-fall assessment tools and the creation of evidence-based fall prevention programs which identifies likely causes for this age group. Since there is no empiric evidence to suggest that fall prevention measures for children are available, hospital staff will need to develop clear policies and procedures based on the policy recommendations from the American Academy of Pediatrics, The U.S. Consumer Product Safety Commission and unintentional fall injury data from the National Center for Injury Prevention and Control Recommendations. Physical restraints may be used in response to children who might be prone to fall or who have fallen in the past. Often application of physical restraints, such as limb restraints, has been used to provide for a level of safety and facilitate diagnostic/therapeutic modalities. Other injury prevention modalities are commonly employed in hospital settings caring for children. Helmets are used often with children known to have seizures. Seizures are associated with head trauma/injury and potential loss of consciousness sustained during a fall. Their use is to prevent traumatic brain injuries arising from skull fractures. Padded side-rails are also used to prevent injury arising from thrashing in bed or from seizing in bed. Hospital policy should be reviewed to determine if bed or chair falls and their prevention are addressed. For instance, does the facility routinely employ use of raised bed-rails on pediatric beds, and if so, are they considered a restraining device? Pediatricians should be consulted to evaluate unexplained or sudden onset of falls in children as part of a plan of care that addresses their diagnosis and management.

Figure 3-7 Essential Domains of the Post-Fall Index
© Deanna Gray-Miceli, DNSc, APRN, FAANP, 2006.

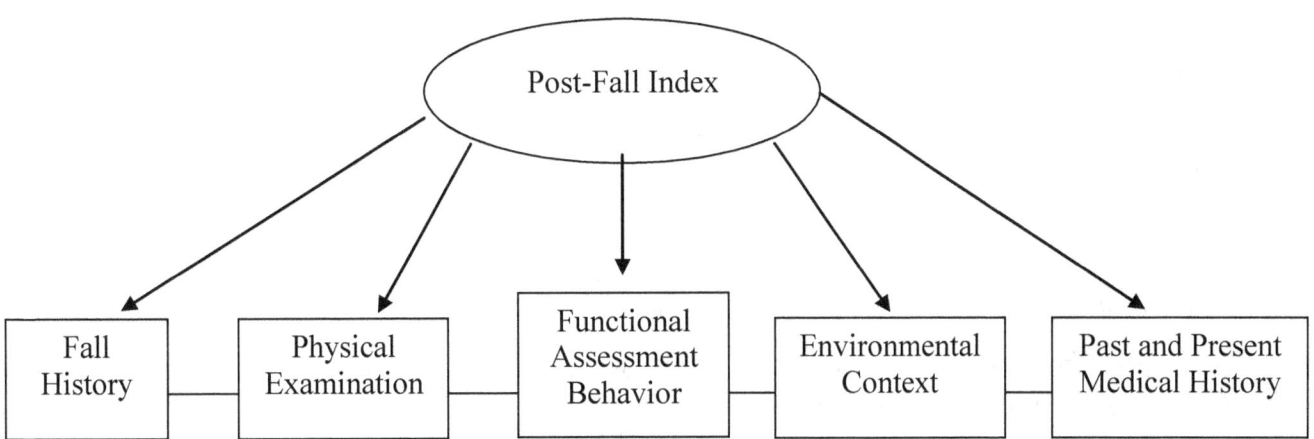

End Notes

[1] Institute of Medicine Report. *To Err is Human: Building a Safer Health System*. National Academy Press, Washington, DC, 2001.

[2] American Geriatrics Society, British Geriatrics Society, American Academy of Orthopedic Surgeons Panel on Falls Prevention. "Guidelines for the prevention of falls in older persons." *Journal of the American Geriatrics Society,* 49(5), pgs. 664-681, 2001.

[3] Moreland, J., Richardson, J., Chan, D.H., et al. "Evidenced-based guidelines for the secondary prevention of falls in older adults", *Gerontology* 49: pgs. 93-116, 2003.

[4] American Medical Directors Association (AMDA) and The American Health Care Association (1998; 2003) *Falls and fall risk: Clinical Practice Guideline*, American Medical Directors Association, Columbia, MD. [Online]. Available on Internet at: http://www.amda.com/clinical/falls/figure_1.htm.

[5] American Academy of Pediatrics Policy (2005). Available on the Internet at: http://aappolicy.aappublications.org/cgi/content/full/pediatrics. Accessed 3/31/07

[6] http: www.cpsc.gov/, The National Center for Injury Prevention and Control [NPIPC] the U.S. Consumer Product Safety Commission

[7] Id.

[8] National SAFE KIDS Campaign available on the Internet at http://www.safekids.org

[9] See note 3.

[10] Firth-Cozens, J. "Cultures for improving patient safety through learning: the role of teamwork," *Quality in Healthcare* 10 (Suppl 11): pgs. 26-31, 2001.

[11] See Note 1.

[12] Reason, J. *Human Error*: New York: Cambridge University Press, 1990.

[13] Joint Commission on Accreditation of Healthcare Organizations. Sentinel event policy and procedures [online]. 2005 June [cited 2006 Feb 10]. Available from Internet: http://www.jcaho.org/accredited+organizations/sentinel+event/se_pp.htm.

[14] Wald, H., and Shojania, K. Chapter 5: "Root cause analysis". [Online]. Available on Internet at: http://www.ahrq.gov/clinic/ptsafety/chap5.htm.

[15] Joint Commission on Accreditation of Healthcare Organizations. Available on the Internet at: http://www.jointcommission.org/NR/rdonlyres/FA5A080F-C259-47CC-AAC8-BAC3F5C. Accessed 3/31/07.

[16] Laska, L. (Ed). "Failure to respond to ring for assistance", *Medical Malpractice Verdicts, Settlements and Experts*, pg. 19, August 2005.

[17] Miceli, D.G., Strumpf, N. E., Reinhard, S. C., Zanna, M. T., & Fritz, E. "Current approaches to post-fall assessment in nursing homes", *Journal of American Medical Directors Association*, 5, pgs. 387-394, 2004.

[18] http://cfrcwww.social.uiuc.edu/LRpdfs/Bruises.LitRev.pdf

[19] Laska, L. (Ed). "Failure to implement fall precautions for elderly patient with mental status change diagnosis", *Medical Malpractice Verdicts, Settlements and Experts*, pg. 19, December 2004.

[20] Laska, L. (Ed). "Collapse during transfer from bed to MRI table blamed for brain damage and lumbar spine injury", *Medical Malpractice Verdicts, Settlements and Experts*, pg. 18, June 2005.

[21] Perell, K. L., Nelson, A., Goldman, R. L., Luther, S. L., Prieto-Lewis, N., & Rubenstein, L. Z. "Fall risk assessment measures: An analytical review." *The Journal of Gerontology*, 56A(12), pgs. M761-M766, 2001.

[22] Id.

[23] "Benching Marking Best Practices Pediatric Benchmarking." [Online]. Available on Internet at: http://www.mmpcorp.com/bench.html.

[24] See Note 17

[25] Gray-Miceli, D., Strumpf, N.E. "Post-Fall Assessment: Development and Validation of a Tool for use with Older Nursing Home Residents". 57th Annual Scientific Meeting of the Gerontological Society of America. *The Gerontologist Program Abstracts* 44, 1, pg.127, 2004.

[26] Gray-Miceli, D., Strumpf, N.E., Johson, J.C., Ratcliffe, S.J. "Psychometric properties of the post-fall index", *Clinical Nursing Research* August, 2006.

[27] Laska, L. (Ed). "Failure to properly monitor resident and respond to calls for help", *Medical Malpractice Verdicts, Settlements and Experts*, pg. 36, February, 2001.

[28] Department of Health and Human Services, Health Care Financing Administration. *Side Rails Guidance*, February 4, 1997.

[29] Ray, W. A., Taylor, J. A., Meador, K. G., Thapa, P. B., Brown, A. K., Kajihara, H. K., et al. "A randomized trial of a consultation service to reduce falls in nursing homes", *Journal of the American Medical Association*, 278, pgs. 557-562, 1997.

[30] Jensen, Lundin-Olsson, Nyberg, & Gustafson, 2002 Jensen, J., Lundin-Olsson, L., Nyberg, L., & Gustafson, Y. "Fall and injury prevention in older people living in residential care facilities: a cluster randomized trial", *Annals of Internal Medicine*, 136, pgs. 733-741, 2002.

[31] Becker, C., Kron, M., Lindermann, U., Sturm, E., Eichner, B., Walter-Jung, B., et al. "Effectiveness of a multifaceted intervention on falls in nursing home residents", *Journal of the American Geriatrics Society*, 51, pgs. 306-313, 2003.

[32] Gillespie et al., Gillespie, L. D., Gillespie, W. J., Robertson, M. C., Lamb, S. E., Cumming, R. G., & Rowe, B. H. "Interventions for preventing falls in the elderly", *Cochrane Database of Systematic Reviews*, 1, 2004.

[33] Van Doorn, C., Gruber-Baldini, A. L., Zimmerman, S., Hebel, J. R., Port, C. L., Baumgarten, M., et al. "Dementia as a risk factor for falls and fall injuries among nursing home residents", *Journal of the American Geriatrics Society*, 51, pgs.1213-1218, 2003.

[34] Patterson, J. E., Strumpf, N. E., & Evans, L. K. "Nursing consultation to reduce restraints in a nursing home", *Clinical Nurse Specialist,* 9, pgs. 231-235, 1995.

[35] Ray, W.A., Taylor, J.A., Meador, K.G., Thapa, P.B., A.K. Kajihara, H.K., et al. "A randomized trial of a consultation service to reduce falls in nursing homes", *Journal of the American Medical Association,* 278, pgs. 557-562, 1997.

[36] Schnelle, J. F., Ouslander, J. G., & Cruise, P. A. "Policy without technology: A barrier to improving nursing home care", *The Gerontologist,* 37, pgs. 527-532, 1997.

[37] Personal communication from Sharon Stahl Wexler, PhD, RN C

[38] Haines, Bennell, & Osborne, Haines, T. P., Bennell, K. L., & Osborne, R. H. "Effectiveness of targeted falls prevention programme in subacute hospital setting: Randomized controlled trial", *British Medical Journal,* 328 pgs. 676-679, 2004.

[39] Healey, Monro & Cockram, Healey, F., Monro, A., & Cockram, A. "Using targeted risk factor reduction to prevent falls in older in-patients: A randomized controlled trial", *Age and Ageing,* 33, pgs. 390-395, 2004.

[40] Edelberg, H. K. "Falls and function. How to prevent falls and injuries in patients with low mobility", *Geriatrics,* 56(3), pgs. 41-45, 49, 2001.

[41] Capezuti, E. "Building the science of falls-prevention research", *Journal of the American Geriatrics Society,* 52, pgs. 461-462, 2004.

[42] Id

[43] Id

[44] Id

Prevention of Falls in Nursing Home Residents
by Elizabeth Capezuti

CHAPTER 4

Chapter 4 Prevention of Falls in Nursing Home Residents

Elizabeth Capezuti, PhD., RN, FAAN

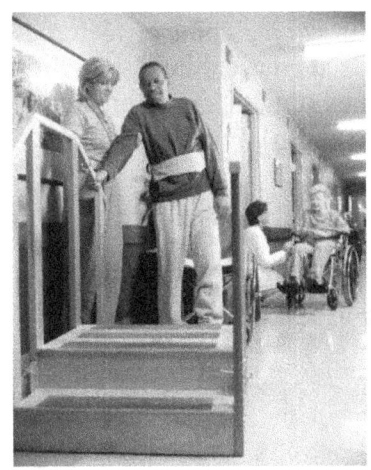

Figure 4-1 "Contact guard" or the therapist's hands on the patient to prevent a fall

A. Federal Regulations

Falls in nursing homes are unique given the specific characteristics of the typical nursing home population, and equipment in use in these facilities. The nursing home industry is heavily regulated; fall prevention is addressed in the federal standards. Federal regulations and their guidance to surveyors point out the standards regarding falls and fractures:

F221 The facility ensures that residents are free from any physical restraints unless they are required to treat the resident's medical symptoms.

F274 The facility provides a timely, prompt assessment after residents experience significant changes in condition.

F309 The facility ensures that each resident receives and the facility provides the necessary care and services to attain or maintain the highest practical physical, mental and psychosocial well-being in accordance with the comprehensive assessment and plan of care.

F323 The facility ensures that the resident environment remains as free of accidents hazards as possible.

F324 The facility must identify each resident at risk for accidents and provide supervision and assistance devices to prevent accidents.

B. Fall Risk Assessment in the Nursing Home

1. The process and use of fall risk assessment tools

The assessment of fall risk is the responsibility of medical, nursing, and rehabilitation staff of the nursing home. Every resident is to be evaluated with the MDS (Minimum Data Set), the RAP (Resident Assessment Protocol) triggers, and when indicated, the RAP Guidelines (all required by Federal regulations).[1] Additionally, a facility (or chain) may have its own fall risk assessment tool and a specific policy and procedure describing its use. Note that fall risk assessment is performed as a screening measure (primary level of prevention) for all residents admitted to a nursing home facility (to detect and modify existing risks to fall), and it is repeated as part of a post fall assessment. (This is the secondary level of prevention - see Chapter 3.)

Although there are numerous published fall risk assessment tools, there is no single tool that is considered "standard" in the nursing home.

Most homes will have a fall assessment tool as part of its nursing or rehabilitation (physical and/or occupational) therapy admission evaluation. Although some falls may be isolated events, most residents who have fallen should have a thorough post-fall assessment (as discussed in Chapter 3). This is especially necessary for those with a history of recurrent falls, since a history of falls is identified as a major risk factor for subsequent falls.[2]

> Critical thinking point for the legal nurse consultant: Does the facility have fall risk assessment tools and separate post-fall assessment tools for evaluation of the falling older adult?

The frequency with which a resident fell is often a factor cited in a malpractice suit.

In *Eggerding v. Chase Nursing Center,* in February of 1998, Erwin Eggerding placed his wife, Nola, age eighty-eight, in the Chase Nursing Center. She suffered from Alzheimer's disease. During her stay, Nola fell some twelve times, sustaining a variety of injuries, including a fractured hip on April 17, 1998. Malnourished, Nola lost thirty-three pounds while at Chase. She also had serious pressure ulcers, particularly on her heels. That complication led to amputation on one leg. Two weeks later she was dead. The jury returned a verdict for the estate, awarding compensatory damages of $500,000, plus another $1,000,000 in punitive damages.[3]

2. Risk factors

An essential aspect of any fall assessment tool is the consideration of risk factors for injurious falls. See below for a list of risk factors that should prompt a thorough evaluation and plan of care.

Figure 4-2 Nursing Home Risk Factors for Falls

Circumstances
- New admission to nursing home
- Recent transfer from hospital or other setting
- Recent transfer from another unit or room
- Responding to bladder or bowel urgency
- Attempting to remove a physical restraint
- Climbing over or around side rails
- History of recurrent falls

Intrinsic

Functional
- Loss of leg or arm movement
- Unilateral (one-sided) weakness
- Recent, rapid decline in functional status (ability to care oneself)

Musculoskeletal
- Arthritis
- Osteoporosis
- History of fracture
- Post-amputation

Neuro-muscular
- Stroke
- Parkinson's disease

Neuro-sensory
- Impaired vision
- Impaired hearing
- Dizziness
- Vertigo
- Polyneuropathy (reduced sensation of extremities) of diabetes, peripheral vascular disease or alcoholism
- Pain, especially of joints

Psychiatric
- Delirium (often indicative of underlying, acute, physical illness)
- Dementia

>   Depression
>
> **Acute illness**
> > Infection
> > Myocardial infarction

Extrinsic
> **Medications**
> > Polypharmacy
> > Cardiac, Antihypertensives, and diuretics
> > Psychoactive
> > > Sedatives, anti-anxiety agents
> > > Benzodiazapines
> > > > Valium
> > > > Chloral hydrate
> > >
> > > Antidepressants
> > > > Tricyclic antidepressants
> > > > Selective serotonin-reuptake inhibitors
> > > > Trazodone
> > >
> > > Antipsychotics
> > > > Haldol

Environmental hazards
> Slippery floors, especially from urine
> Glare from highly polished floors
> Absence of night lights
> Unstable furniture
> Low chairs without armrest support or seat back
> Low toilet seats without secure gab bars

Assistive devices
> Wheelchair
> Walker
> Cane, especially if poorly maintained or not fitted properly to the individual resident's size and needs
> Physical restraints, including side rails

Behavioral
> Risk-taker personality or impulsive mobility (may be secondary to stroke or impaired cognition)
> Tendency to stand quickly, especially from bed or immediately after a meal

Sources: Centers for Medicare and Medicaid Services (2002). *Resident assessment protocols. Centers for Medicare and Medicaid RAI Version 2.0 Manual* (Appendix C, 1-4, 59-62). Grisso, J. A., Capezuti, E., & Schwartz, A. (1996). Falls as risk factors for fractures. In R. Arcus, D. Feldman and J. Kelsey (Eds.). *Osteoporosis*. San Diego: Academic Press

The failure to adequately assess fall risk in nursing home residents and to develop and follow a specific care plan has also been held to be a deviation from the standard of care, and is a basis for the imposition of liability.

In *Debbie Johnson, Individually and as Administratix of the Estate of Pearl Bean, deceased; Marie Cruse; and Richard Bean v. S.C.T.W. Health Care Center, Inc.*, the three adult children of the decedent brought suit after their mother was allowed to fall five times in the Bayou Pines Nursing

Home over a twenty-seven-day period in 1999. The fifth fall resulted in a fractured neck and multiple rib fractures which the plaintiffs claimed caused her death. The plaintiffs contended that prior to decedent's admission to the nursing home, the staff conducted a pre-admission assessment in which it was specifically noted that she "falls easily and has a history of numerous falls." Unfortunately, the in-home assessment was not provided to the admitting nurse at Bayou Pines, nor was the information included in her chart at the facility. Other alleged significant established failures included the nurses' disregard of a physician's order to obtain a physical therapy evaluation, the failure to perform a fall risk evaluation, and the failure to follow the care plan. This action settled for $1,000,000. [4]

C. Addressing Side Effects of Medications

A variety of medications are associated with increased fall risk. A pharmacy consultant is required to review the medications of each resident and make written recommendations to the resident's attending physician. This review is meant to uncover potential drug-drug interactions and to make suggestions regarding inappropriate drug usage. The MDS contains a "seven day look back" at the number and types of medications administered to each resident (section O of the MDS). Additionally, as part of the RAP Guidelines for Falls, the multidisciplinary clinical team should consider the role of medications in causing a fall in a resident. Examples of specific guidelines questions are: (1) Were medications, known to cause related problems (low blood pressure, rigid muscles, tremors or decreased alertness), administered prior to or after the fall, and (2) If administered prior to the fall, how close to the incident were they given?

All psychoactive drugs have been implicated in increasing fall risk. Psychoactive drugs include anti-psychotics, sedatives (sleeping pills), anti-anxiety drugs and antidepressants. [5,6,7] In October 1990, implementation of the OBRA '87 mandate to reduce psychoactive medication use in nursing homes was begun. The regulations provide detailed guidelines regarding the prescription of these medications and indicate that these drugs should be used only to treat specific illnesses and not behavioral symptoms such as wandering, combativeness, or lack of cooperation. A drug used for non-medical purposes such as discipline or convenience would be "tagged" as a deficiency as use of a "chemical restraint." The significant reduction of psychoactive drug use in nursing homes post-OBRA is well documented. [8,9]

According to OBRA '87, psychoactive medications (anti-psychotics, anti-anxiety or hypnotics, and anti-depressants) may only be prescribed for specific psychiatric diagnoses (e.g., schizophrenia) and not for dementia (also known as organic brain syndrome). In fact, the use of psychoactive medications to control behavior is considered a type of "chemical restraint." The medication dosage must not exceed the recommended 24-hour limit; an attempt must be made to reduce the dosage or use of antipsychotic medications in those taking them for six months or more. [10] Medication side effects must be carefully monitored. For example, in addition to increasing fall risk, some anti-psychotic medications can result in symptoms of Parkinson's disease. These symptoms, which include tremors and muscle rigidity, have been shown to increase fall risk and warrant immediate discontinuation of the medication. [11] Further research into medications and fall-risk will help in treating the elderly and their numerous co-morbidities without increasing fall rates.

The RAP for Psychotropic Drug Use assists nursing home staff in carefully evaluating the indications for use and promotes discontinuation of psychoactive drugs causing problematic side effects, including falls. Every fall case, therefore, requires a thorough review of medication (especially psychoactive drug) use.

Critical thinking point for the legal nurse consultant: Is there evidence in the patient's medical record or in the plan of care that a medication was lowered, substituted, or discontinued if recommended by the pharmacist.

D. Providing Appropriate Observation

Call bells are meant to inform the nursing staff when a resident needs assistance. Many nursing home residents, however, are unable to use call bells due to cognitive or physical impairments. New "bulb" call bells, sensitive to very light pressure, are more easily used by those with arthritic hands or those experiencing weakness from a stroke or other neuromuscular disorder.

Critical thinking point: Is there documentation or evidence that the call light was placed in an accessible position for the resident, especially if the resident had a unilateral hemiparesis limiting use of one of the arms? Did the facility management institute call bell safety checks during environmental rounds to ensure proper functioning?

Periodic observation of the resident is a basic intervention to prevent falls. Staff should evaluate whether a resident is participating in an activity that could lead to a fall (e.g. walking without a prescribed cane) or needs assistance such as help with getting to the bathroom. [12]

It is customary to expect that every resident is observed at least every two hours.

Some nursing home staff have checklists or make notations in the nurses' or CNAs' (certified nursing assistant) shift notes of "Seen on Q2H (every two hours) rounds." However, studies of compliance with these rounds, despite documentation of Q2H rounds, have shown that this is rarely enforced. [13,14] If the facility has a documented policy for "Q2H" rounds, but it is not implemented in practice, this may leave the facility open to liability. Policies and procedures are expected to follow national standards of practice. Documentation of staff's adherence to these policies should not be vague. For example, notes documenting the exact times the resident was observed and his or her position/condition with the staff member's initials or signature are better indicators of compliance.

Observation may be facilitated by placing the resident in an area near a nursing station or in a multi-purpose "day" or dining room where a staff member is present or can view the room easily from a nurses' station. Some homes use video monitors to view the "day" room or resident rooms. This latter practice may be questionable due to its potential violation of resident privacy rights. Appropriate supervision of residents should be provided.

Critical thinking point for the legal nurse consultant: Did the facility provide a room monitor to observe and assist residents who may need to get up from their chairs to urinate? If yes, is there documentation of this?

In *Boren v. DeKalb Medical Center and Christian Towers,* the plaintiff was a 90-year-old widowed female who was a resident of the defendant Christian Towers facility. A group of residents were being transported by van to the defendant Medical Center when the plaintiff fell and suffered a hairline fracture to her hip. The driver of the van, employed by Christian Towers, had left the building to pull the van up when the incident occurred. One week after injury, the plaintiff fell in her apartment. She subsequently underwent surgery on her hip and then suffered a stroke.

The defendants received summary judgments in their favor which were appealed by the plaintiff. The Court of Appeals upheld the summary judgment in favor of the Medical Center—but reversed the summary judgment for Christian Towers. The plaintiff alleged that the defendant Towers' employee left the plaintiff in the building without assistance required for her supervision and ambulation and that the defendant Towers was responsible for the negligence of its employee. The plaintiff also maintained that the falls, surgery, and stroke were all related to the original incident as described. The jury awarded the plaintiff $16,000. [15]

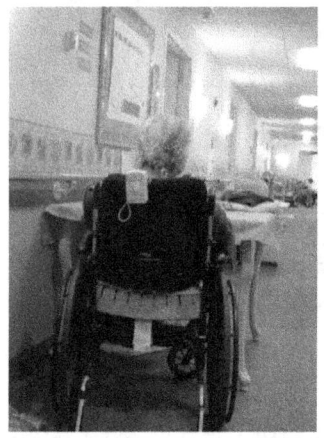

Figure 4-2 Chair Alarm

A variety of bed and chair-exit alarms (Figure 4-3) can help to monitor the activities of residents and maintain a restraint-free environment, though they require staff vigilance and assistance. Alarms can be pressure-sensitive (an alarm sounds when the resident lifts his/her buttocks off sensor pad; see Figure 4-4) or may sound when the resident attempts to stand (sensor on thigh). Also an alarm unit can be attached to the bed or chair and a clip attached to the resident's clothing; the alarm will sound when the sensor is disconnected from a central unit. Note that patients may remove or disconnect their personal alarm because of annoyance or failure to recall its intended purpose (such as in the case of individuals who have judgment or memory impairment). If repeated removal of a personal alarm occurs, re-assessment of the patient and plan of care is immediately warranted, while other interventions for fall prevention are instituted. Other alarms include pressure-sensitive floor mats placed next to the bed and infrared beam detectors which are activated when the beam is broken by the resident attempting to exit the bed. [16] A number of small studies have shown that alarms can decrease incidence of falls and may be used as an effective prevention method. However, a July 2001 Agency for Health Care Policy and Research (AHRQ) report analyzing many of the studies on bed-exit alarms found insufficient evidence about their effectiveness in preventing falls. They conclude that further research is warranted before recommending bed-exit alarm use in clinical practice.

In *Lynn Pascarelli, Administratrix for the Estate of Helen Whitaker v. Frontier of Connecticut,* an 84-year-old double amputee was a resident in the defendant Connecticut nursing home. She fell from her bed at the home, fracturing her nose, injuring her neck and back, and suffering a periorbital edema. She subsequently died of unrelated causes. Her administratrix contended that the decedent routinely moved down her bed as she slept, that bed sensors and bed alarms were the standard of care, and that their use would have prevented the fall from occurring. The defendant argued that bed sensors and bed alarms were not the standard of care, that side rails were in place, and that their staff did everything they were required to do to prevent the fall. According to the Verdict Reporter, the verdict was for the defense. [17]

ECRI (formerly the Emergency Care Research Institute) is a non-profit health services research agency which conducts much needed research in this area. In May 2004, ECRI published an important article guiding practitioners on the use of bed-exit alarms as an "early warning system" to alert staff when residents attempt to leave their bed unassisted. [18] They emphasize that the alarms themselves do not prevent falls and must be carefully utilized as one component of a comprehensive falls prevention program. Despite a lack of clinical data, Joint Commission endorses the use of bed alarms and proposes them as a means of reducing the risk of falls and fall-related injuries. [19]

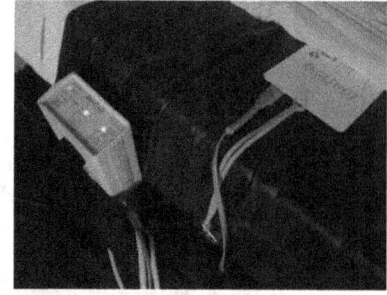

> *Critical thinking point for the legal nurse consultant:* Examine capital costs and expenses for fall prevention aids for a particular nursing home. Can you determine if bed-or chair alarms were purchased by the facility? If there were no purchases for such devices, can you determine if the policy and procedural manual addresses private duty nursing, one-to-one personal assistance, or other resources for fall prevention?

In *Anonymous Nursing Home Resident v. Anonymous Nursing Home*, the plaintiff was in a nursing home for thirty-three days in 1997. She alleged that within two weeks of her short admission to this facility, she fell five times. The plaintiff's last fall at the nursing home on September 27, 1997 caused her to suffer an intraventricular bleed, after which she was admitted to the hospital for five days. The plaintiff's spouse signed a consent form for installation of side rail restraints while the patient was in her bed. A TABS alarm monitor was initiated. The monitor is designed to alert the staff when the patient may be moving from side-to-side in the edge of the bed, or rising off of a chair seat. On the day of the last fall, the nurse's notes stated, "Found patient lying face down on the floor by the bottom of the bed this a.m. TABS alarm was removed from her clothing. Resident sustained 7 by 5 centimeter bump with an ecchymosis of her left forehead." After investigation and discovery, it was determined that the bed rails may not have been up, and that the TABS alarm never sounded. It was not until fifty-four hours after the injury and fall that the resident, on the request of the family, was sent to the hospital for evaluation. A complaint was filed with the Department of Public Health regarding the falls and treatment of the resident. The DPH investigation revealed that the nursing home failed to modify the care plan in light of the falls. The investigation questioned why a low bed with floor padding had not been considered for this resident. The DPH issued a deficiency as a result of its findings. It was noted by the DPH investigation report that the TABS monitor was not attached properly as per the manufacturer's instructions, and the facility failed to educate the staff on proper installation. This action resulted in a $125,000 settlement, according to a published account.[20]

Elopement control devices work similarly to department store tag devices. An identification tag placed on the resident's wrist or ankle will signal the detection monitoring device when the resident walks by it, thus, setting off the alarm.[21] These devices are used for wanderers who may walk into unsafe areas of the nursing home or outside, potentially sustaining a fall and/or injury.

> In order for any alarm system to facilitate fall prevention it must be in good working order; these devices are known to break down frequently.

Some of these alarms, such as the pressure-sensitive and position-changing devices, require adjustment of the delay time. This is the amount of time between the resident's change in position and sounding of the alarm. If the delay is too short, there will be frequent false alarms that will annoy both the resident and the staff; if too long, there will be inadequate time for the staff to reach the resident.

> All alarm systems depend on the ability of staff to reach the resident in a timely manner. If the resident is located far from staff, no alarm may be adequate.

New alarms include a voice alarm - a tape recorder that can play an individualized message addressing the resident by name and calmly instructing the resident to remain in his/her chair until the nurse arrives to provide assistance. Unfortunately, lack of staff is still a reality at many nursing homes and may pose safety code violations placing residents at risk and undermining fall prevention measures. As of January 1, 2003, CMS required nursing homes to publicly post numbers of licensed and unlicensed nursing staff numbers for each shift who provide resident care. Complaints, deficiencies, and MDS data (on falls, weight loss, etc) can all be used to analyze whether an investigation into inadequate staffing is warranted.

E. Promoting Safe Mobility

Among those who have some ability or potential to walk ("ambulatory"), most falls occur while ambulating. Many residents may have preserved gait skills and be able to ambulate quickly, but have impaired balance skills, presenting a particularly high-risk combination for falls. [22] A thorough evaluation of gait and balance disturbances is necessary, especially considering most disturbances are treatable and improved mobility will likely lead to a reduced likelihood of falls. [23] In 1990, the National Institutes of Health sponsored eight clinical trials concerning physical frailty and fall-related injuries of older persons called FICSIT (Frailty and Injuries: Cooperative Studies of Intervention Techniques). [24] Physical frailty, defined as "severely impaired strength, mobility, balance and endurance" is viewed as the chief factor responsible for increasing the likelihood of falls and injuries. [25] The FICSIT intervention studies conducted with a sample of frail nursing home residents, found that muscle strengthening exercises can improve function and reduce falls. [26] This study and others [27,28] supports the use of rehabilitation and restorative nursing programs in nursing homes, though some trials of exercise programs alone question their effectiveness in preventing falls. [29]

Rehabilitation includes physical and/or occupational therapy aimed at improving joint mobility and muscle strengthening, along with prescription and education of correct usage of assistive devices for walking, sitting, or lying in bed. Every nursing home resident must be screened by both physical and occupational therapy at the time of admission. The revised MDS includes an objective performance-based measure of ambulation (section G), such as farthest distance walked, support provided while ambulating, and so on, but does not yet include measures of balance.

Resident preferences about level of mobility should be respected.

In a nursing home, an 85-year-old female had self-care and mobility deficits related to a diagnosis of progressive supra nuclear palsy (SNP). The SNP was profound with associated gait ataxia, speech difficulties and impaired communication. Each time the patient stood, she fell, an average of over ten times per day. She was diagnosed with osteoporosis in addition to the SNP. She was usually in good spirits and was visited frequently by her children and friends. Her children requested physical restraint use, which was denied, but shared decision-making and frank discussion about the potential for injury such as fractured bones or head injury lead to her decision to travel by wheel-chair. Although her decisional-capacity for complex issues was impaired, she was still able to make some simple choices about walking. This choice appeared to be the most appropriate given the nature of her progressive SNP and the high potential for a serious injury and most consistent with a principle of selecting the least restrictive option (i.e, evidence-based practice to avoid use of physical restraints).

Critical thinking point for the legal nurse consultant: Did the facility offer through its physical therapy department a generalized or lower extremity exercise program for older adults who were wheelchair bound, but retained lower extremity strength and function?

If a resident falls, the RAP for falls requires a thorough evaluation addressing modifiable risk factors. The resident with recurrent or injurious falls should be evaluated by a physical or occupational therapist. The therapist's recommendations should then be discussed in a multi-disciplinary care conference and documented in the MDS quarterly assessment or the interdisciplinary plan of care. Recommendations may include use of an assistive device such as a leg brace, cane or walker. Such devices should be individualized to the resident's height and abilities.

Rehabilitative or restorative nursing care refers to walking programs, range of motion (exercise of joints), and other activities conducted by nursing or physical therapy assistants that have been prescribed by a physical/occupational therapist, nurse or physiatrist (physician specializing in physical medicine and rehabilitation). The purpose of these activities is to maintain function and prevent adverse complications due to immobilization such as contractures (joint permanently or temporarily fixed or immobile) and pressure ulcers.

Critical thinking point for the legal nurse consultant: Does the facility train staff such as nurse's aides to walk older adult residents on a daily basis to preserve mobility?

Environmental factors to prevent falls include uncluttered walkways free of furniture or small objects that can block the path in the hallways, dining room, "day" room and, most importantly, the bedroom. Proper lighting is especially important to nursing home residents who often have visual impairments. At night, low-voltage lights as well as lights that are easy to turn on or automatically illuminate with motion can help prevent nighttime falls.

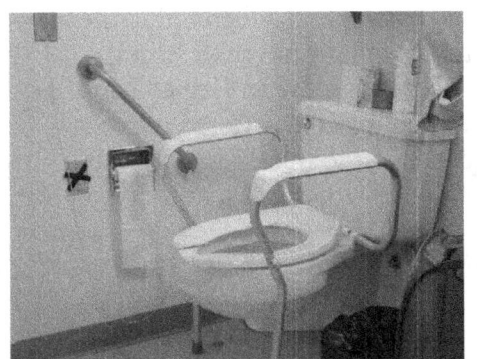

F. Promoting Safe Transferring

In addition to falling while walking, ambulatory residents often fall when attempting to transfer to and from bed, chair, or toilet. (See figure 4-5.) Among those unable to walk ("non-ambulatory"), most injurious falls occur when staff attempts to transfer residents. Thus, improving the safety of transferring skills is important to fall prevention.[30] Bed height (the distance between the floor and the top of the mattress) is crucial to safe standing. For shorter (less than five feet) residents, the bed may be too high for safe transfer. Low beds are now available that can be manually, hydraulically or electrically adjusted to promote transfer.[31] A non-skid mat placed at the side of the bed and/or toilet can reduce the likelihood of slipping.[32] In the bathroom, securely fastened grab bars, as well as a toilet seat individually adjusted to the resident's height, will reduce falls in the bathroom. An emergency call light must be present and in working order. Periodic safety checks of this device are important.

CNAs must partially or completely assist residents with no physical or cognitive (e.g. severe Alzheimer's disease) ability to transfer safely. Some injurious falls may be due to improper transfer techniques by the CNAs.

In *Yannelli and Wolfstern v. Methodist Hospital Nursing Center,* the plaintiff's mother was staying in the defendant Pennsylvania nursing center. She suffered a fractured tibia and fibula while being transferred from a chair to a bed. The plaintiff alleged that the defendant's employees used improper transfer techniques to move her. The patient's leg had to be placed in a cast. When the cast was removed, a compound fracture of the leg was discovered, and part of her skin stuck to the cast. The woman underwent surgery for the compound fracture and subsequently developed bed sores. She died before the start of trial. According to a published account, the defendant admitted liability at trial. The jury returned a $250,000 verdict for the plaintiff. [33]

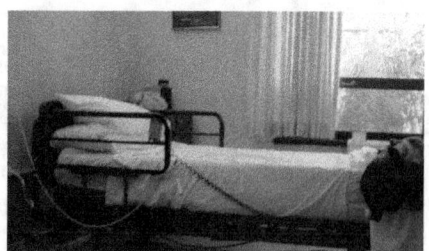

Figure 4-5 A Low Rise Bed Minimizes Distance from the Mattress to the Floor

The nursing home may be liable if the care plan documents that transferring the resident from bed to chair requires two persons or one person with a Hoyer lift but one CNA transfers and drops a resident without the lift. A Hoyer lift is a device that one or two persons can use to assist with moving an overweight or very weak person (such as a person who has had a stroke, Parkinson's disease, or spinal cord injury.) It includes a sling that can be placed under the resident's buttocks or around the waist or shoulders. The sling is attached to a hydraulic lift that raises or lowers the resident. This device should only be used by a nurse or CNA with proper training in the use of the device in general and with the individual resident specifically. The sling needs to be properly washed and dried to avoid damage from high heat or bleach. Inspection of the sling for tears or fraying should be performed before its use with the Hoyer lift.

Critical thinking point for the legal nurse consultant: Did the facility regularly train staff in correct handling techniques, transferring patient and body mechanics?

In *Jane Doe v. Roe Convalescent Hospital,* a 76-year-old woman was being transferred from her bed to a wheelchair by employees of the defendant convalescent hospital. As she was being lifted, the Hoyer lift failed that was being used to pick up and move her. The plaintiff then fell to the ground and was severely injured. The plaintiff contended that the hospital was reckless in its maintenance of the Hoyer lift. The plaintiff sustained multiple fractures of the left leg and an intraarticular fracture with malunion of the left leg. She also claimed that she suffered pressure sores, skin damage, and diminished health due to inactivity because of the fractures. She also sustained aggravation of arthritis in the left leg, as well as emotional distress and fear of losing her left leg. The plaintiff settled her case for $425,000. [34]

G. Promoting Comfortable, Individualized Seating

Falls in the nursing home often occur when a resident slides out of a chair, "flips" a chair, or attempts to unsafely rise from an uncomfortable chair.

There are numerous chairs and devices on the market that fulfill a variety of resident needs. For example, glider or rocking chairs with vinyl-covered cushions are used with residents who like to rock and have a tendency to fall forward out of a wheelchair or stationary chair. Recliners without tray tables can be a comfortable alternative to a chair, however, they often require additional cushions to promote correct and comfortable positioning.

Critical thinking point for the legal-nurse consultant: Were there a variety of chair-types, thereby adding customization to patient needs? Analyze of the types of chairs purchased by the nursing facility.

> Remaining in a reclining position for most of the day will eventually result in the decreased ability to sit up in a wheelchair or straight back chair due to loss of abdominal muscle strength. This will adversely affect the resident's ability to eat or swallow liquids safely (without aspiration). Treatment of weak abdominal muscles usually requires a process of incrementally reducing the angle of recline over time; and supervision of this process is done by an occupational therapist.

Most nursing home residents spend the majority of the day and early evening hours in a wheelchair. Wheelchairs were originally designed for transport; their sling seats do not provide adequate support for long periods of sitting. Many products are available to adapt the chair to the resident's seating needs.[35] If the resident spends more than an hour per day in a wheelchair or hard plastic/wood chair, the chair should, at minimum, have some type of pressure-relieving seat cushion. Anti-tippers applied to chair will prevent the resident from "flipping" a wheelchair or chair forward or backward.

Other adaptations for the wheelchair include a wedge cushion inserted under the resident's buttocks and thighs which tilt the resident backward. A wedge seat prevents the resident from sliding forward. Similarly, leaning to the side is corrected with lateral supports or cushions. Stroke victims with hemiplegia (one-sided weakness) are at risk for shoulder subluxation (partial dislocation) if the weakened arm slips off the side of the chair. This can be prevented with devices attached to a wheelchair: an arm trough, elevated armrest, lateral arm support, or half tray. A full tray table is not necessary. A leg panel will prevent legs from falling backward off foot pedals or between calf pads. A head extension can be added to a wheelchair, or other chairs, to help keep the resident's head erect and promote comfort. Also, "wingback" head extensions will prevent the resident's head from leaning to one side.

The wheelchair itself can be individually fitted to the resident's size. For example, pediatric wheelchairs are available for very small residents as are extra-wide chairs for obese or larger residents. "Walking" in the wheelchair (i.e., using feet to propel forward or backward) is easier for some residents than pushing the wheels with their arms. Hemi-height wheelchairs that can be adjusted to the resident's lower leg length can facilitate pushing the wheelchair with the legs. This adjustment creates safe transport while promoting muscle strengthening exercise to the lower extremities.[36]

> ***Critical thinking point for the legal nurse consultant***: Given the patient's height and body weight, was the chair an appropriate size? If the older adult slides out of the chair, it may be too big or fail to have proper pillow supports. Was the foot rest utilized, which can help reduce the chances of slippage from the chair seat? Was the patient wearing shoes or anti-skid slippers while sitting in the chair?

The need for all of the adaptive equipment described can be determined by a physical/occupational therapist, nurse or physiatrist with the attending physician's orders. Individualized seating, however, is only part of the solution to prevent falls. Residents need regular exercise. No matter how comfortable the chair, residents need to get up periodically. Those unable to move themselves should receive assistance of the staff in changing positions and, if possible, in standing or walking at least twice a day as part of a rehabilitation or restorative nursing program. Also, because sitting up can be tiresome, residents may need to nap for one to two hours in the early afternoon, depending on their condition.

> Some residents will attempt to get up from even the most comfortable chair because of boredom. A stimulating activities program is an important part of a falls prevention program. Also, an activity apron or half tray with an activity board can be help to stimulate the resident with dementia. [37]

H. Preventing Falls from Bed

Most falls from bed occur when transferring in or out of bed. In addition to the aforementioned adjustment of bed height, many residents need a device to enable or assist them in safely transferring out of /into bed. A trapeze may be helpful, however, it requires full shoulder mobility and adequate upper extremity strength. Transfer enablers (transfer pole or bar), or be raised ¼" or ½" length side rails directly attached to or adjacent to the top of the bed promote stability when standing. [38] Another method of preventing falls from bed is to provide reminders to the resident of the bed's perimeters. This may include bed bumpers on mattress edges, concave mattresses, pillows, and other cues to demarcate the bed's perimeter. [39]

> Reducing the risk of injury is paramount for residents with a history of climbing around or over side rails, especially those at high risk of injury.

A very low bed height is recommended for those residents unable to stand safely, but who may accidentally roll out of or attempt to unsafely exit from bed. Most standard nursing home beds can be adjusted to approximately twenty-one inches off the floor. For those at high risk of injury and with a known history of unsafe behavior, it may be necessary to place the mattress directly on the floor or use very low height beds (between seven and thirteen inches above the floor including the mattress.) [40] Also, beds are available that can be adjusted manually, electrically or hydraulically from a few inches off the floor to twenty-six inches. [41] The ability to adjust the bed height to at least twenty-six inches is preferred since this can prevent staff back injuries.

Falling onto a hard surface increases the likelihood of serious injury. [42] Thus, specialized flooring such as carpet or a bedside cushion such as an exercise mat or an eggcrate foam mattresses is useful for those at risk of fall-related injury. [43] Also, the use of hip-protector pads has been shown to reduce the risk of hip fracture in nursing home fallers. [44,45,46,47] While hip protectors should be utilized as an important prevention strategy, as is advocated by the AHCPR, issues of compliance with wearing hip protectors remains a barrier to practice. [48]

Promoting comfort and maintaining continence are paramount to the falls prevention effort. [49] Individualized interventions may include nighttime toileting rounds, adequate pain control, and treatment of depression and sleep disorders. [50] In particular situations such as intravenous therapy administration where a resident may be likely to disrupt the treatment, the least restrictive measure should be used rather than potentially hazardous restraints. For example, mittens may be used to prohibit finger movement. Residents may be distracted by an activity such as music or reading magazines. [51]

Falls among older adults in nursing homes can be prevented when known risk factors are reduced and underlying causes identified through a comprehensive fall evaluation. Healthcare providers, staff, and professionals must institute interventions linked to underlying causes and associated risks for each resident, continually evaluating and re-evaluating their effectiveness for fall prevention. The providers must also consider the need to maintain the resident's dignity, autonomy, independence, safety and often times, personal preference. Through an integrated and coordinated team approach focusing on individualized assessment and management, inclusive of the residents and their families, fall prevention interventions are successful. Failure to provide adequate care in these areas of fall prevention and management can lead to litigation, particularly when falls are not resolved or when they result in personal serious injury or fatality.

End notes

[1] Hawes, C., Mor, V., Phillips, C.D., Fries, B.E., Morris, J.N., Steele-Friedlob, E., Greene, A.M., Nennstiel, M. "The OBRA-87 nursing home regulations and implementation of the Residents Assessment Instrument: effects on process quality", *Journal of the American Geriatrics Society*, 45 (8), pgs. 977-985, 1997.

[2] Chang, JT., Morton, SC, Rubenstein, LZ, Mojica, WA, Maglione, M., Suttorp, MJ., Roth, EA and Shekelle, PG. "Interventions for the prevention of falls in older adults: a systematic review and meta-analysis of randomized clinical trials", *British Medical Journal* 20: 328 (7441): 680, 2004.

[3] Laska, L. (Ed). "Alzheimer's patient dies after amputation of leg due to development of pressure ulcers", *Medical Malpractice Verdicts, Settlements and Experts*, pg. 31, February, 2003.

[4] Laska, L. (Ed). "Failure to note patient's propensity for falling", *Medical Malpractice Verdicts, Settlements and Experts*, pg. 41, November, 2002.

[5] Thapa, P. B., Gideon, P., Cost, T. W., Milam, A. B., & Ray, W. A. "Antidepressant and the risk of falls among nursing home residents." *New England Journal of Medicine,* 339, pgs. 875-882, 1998.

[6] Thapa, P. B., Gideon, P., Fought, R. L., et al. "Psychotropic drugs and risk of recurrent falls in ambulatory nursing home residents", *American Journal of Epidemiology,* 142, pgs. 202-211, 1995.

[7] Tinetti, M. E. "Preventing falls in elderly persons: clinical practice", *New England Journal of Medicine,* 348 (1), pgs. 42-49, 2003.

[8] Schorr, R. I., Fought, R. L., & Ray, W. A. "Changes in antipsychotic drug use in nursing homes during implementation of the OBRA'87 regulations", *Journal of the American Medical Association,* 271, pgs.358-362, 1994.

[9] Siegler, E. L., Capezuti, E., Maislin, G., et al. "Effect of a restraint reduction intervention and OBRA '87 regulations on psychoactive drug use in nursing homes", *Journal of the American Geriatrics Society,* 45, pgs. 791-796, 1997

[10] Llorente, M. D., Olsen, E. J., Leyva, O., et al. "Use of antipsychotic drugs in nursing homes: Current compliance with OBRA regulations", *Journal of the American Geriatrics Society,* 46, pgs. 198-201, 1998.

[11] Kalish, S. C., Bohn, R. L., Mogun, H., et al. "Antipsychotic prescribing patterns and the treatment of extrapyramidal symptoms in older people", *Journal of the American Geriatrics Society,* 43, pgs. 967-973, 1995.

[12] Turkoski, B., Pierce, L. L., Schreck, S., et al. "Clinical nursing judgment related to reducing the incidence of falls by elderly patients", *Rehabilitation Nursing,* 22, pgs. 124-129, 1997.

[13] Cruise, P. A., Schnelle, J. F., Alessi, C.A., et al. "The nighttime environment and incontinence care practices in nursing homes", *Journal of the American Geriatrics Society,* 46, pgs. 181-186, 1998.

[14] Schnelle, J. F., Cruise, P. A., Alessi, C. A., et al. "Individualizing nighttime incontinence care in nursing home residents", *Nursing Research,* 47, pgs.197-204, 1998.

[15] Laska, L. (Ed). "Unsupervised elderly resident fractures hip requiring surgery", *Medical Malpractice Verdicts, Settlements and Experts*, pg.36, October, 2002.

[16] "ECRI. Guidance article: bed-exit alarms: a component (but only a component) of fall prevention", *Health Devices, 33,* pgs. 157-168, 2004. Also available: http://www.ecri.org/Newsroom/Document_Details.aspx?docid=20040624_129

[17] Laska, L. (Ed). "Elderly Connecticut woman falls from bed in nursing home", *Medical Malpractice Verdicts, Settlements and Experts,* pg.32, April, 2003.

[18] See note 16.

[19] Joint Commission on Accreditation of Healthcare Organizations. Sentinel event policy and procedures [online]. 2005 June [cited 2006 Feb 10]. Available from Internet: http://www.jcaho.org/accredited+organizations/sentinel+event/se_pp.htm.

[20] Laska, L. (Ed). "Resident identified as at high risk for falls suffers repeated falls during one-month admission", *Medical Malpractice Verdicts, Settlements and Experts,* pg. 31, November, 2003.

[21] Sanford, J. A., Fazenbaker, S. H., & Rose, C. B. "Alarm system technology in elopement prevention", *Technology and Disability*, 2, pgs. 22-33, 1993.

[22] Harrison, B., Booth, D., & Algase, D. "Studying fall risk factors among nursing home residents who fell", *Journal of Gerontological Nursing*, 27(10), pgs. 26-34, 2001.

[23] Rubenstein, L. Z., Powers, C. M., & MacLean, C. H. "Quality indicators for the management and prevention of falls and mobility problems in vulnerable elders", *Annals of Internal Medicine,* 135, pgs. 686-693, 2001.

[24] Ory, M. G., Schectman, K. B., Miller, J. P. et al. "Frailty and injuries in later life: The FICSIT Trials", *Journal of the American Geriatrics Society,* 41, pgs. 283-296, 1993.

[25] Id

[26] Fiatarone, M. A., O'Neil, E. F., Ryan, N. D., et al. "Exercise training and nutritional supplementation for physical frailty in very elderly people", *The New England Journal of Medicine,* 330, pgs. 1769-1775, 1994.

[27] MacRae, P. G., Asplund, L. A., Schnelle, J. F., et al. "A walking program for nursing home residents: Effects on walk endurance, physical activity, mobility, and quality of life." *Journal of the American Geriatrics Society,* 44, pgs. 175-180, 1996.

[28] Shaw, E., & Kenny, R. A. "Can falls in patients with dementia be prevented?" *Age and Ageing*, 27, pgs.7-9, 1998.

[29] Nowalk, M. P., Prendergast, J. M., Bayles, C. M., D'Amico, F. J., & Colvin, G. C. "A randomized trial of exercise programs among older individuals living in two long-term care facilities: the falls free program", *Journal of the American Geriatrics Society,* 49, pgs. 859-865, 2001.

[30] Thapa, P. B., Brockman, K. G., Gideon, P., et al. "Injurious falls in nonambulatory nursing home residents: A comparative study of circumstances, incidence, and risk factors", *Journal of the American Geriatrics Society,* 44, pgs. 273-278, 1996.

[31] Capezuti, L. "Legal liability issues and physical restraints." *HCFA's National Restraint Reduction Newsletter,* 5(3), pgs. 1-2, 9, 1997.

[32] Capezuti, E., Talerico, K. A., Strumpf, N., & Evans, L. "Individualized assessment and intervention in bilateral side rail use", *Geriatric Nursing,* 19, pgs.322-330, 1998.

[33] Laska, L. (Ed) "Pennsylvania nursing home resident suffers broken leg during transfer from chair to bed", *Medical Malpractice Verdicts, Settlements and Experts,* pg.34, May, 2003.

[34] Laska, L. (Ed). "Hoyer lift fails during bed to wheelchair transfer", *Medical Malpractice Verdicts, Settlements and Experts,* pg.36, August, 2003.

[35] Rader, J., Jones, D., and Miller, L. "The importance of individualized wheelchair seating for frail older adults", *Journal of Gerontological Nursing*, 26, pgs.24-32, 2000.

[36] Simmons, S. F., Schnelle, J. F., MacRae, P. G., et al. "Wheelchairs a mobility restraints: Predictors of wheelchair activity in nonambulatory nursing home residents", *Journal of the American Geriatrics Society* 43, pgs. 384-388, 1995.

[37] Strumpf, N. E., Robinson, J. P., Wagner, J. S., et al. *Restraint-free Care.* New York: Springer, 1998.

[38] Capezuti, E., Talerico, K. A., Strumpf, N., & Evans, L. "Individualized assessment and intervention in bilateral side rail use", *Geriatric Nursing, 19*, pgs.322-330, 1998

[39] Capezuti, E., & Wexler, S. S "Choosing alternatives to restraints." In E. L. Siegler, S. Mirafzali, & J. B. Foust (Eds.), *An Introduction to Hospitals and Inpatient Care* (pp. 101-113). New York: Springer, 2003.

[40] Rader, J. Jones, D. & Miller, LL. "Creating a supportive environment for eliminating restraints" In J. Rader and E.M. Tornquist (Eds.). *Individual Dementia Care.* New York: Springer, 1995.

[41] Id.

[42] Nevitt, M. C., & Cummings, S. R. "Type of fall and risk of hip and wrist fracture: The study of osteoporotic fractures", *Journal of the American Geriatrics Society*, 41, pgs.1226-1234, 1993.

[43] Donald, I. P., Pitt, K., Armstrong, E., & Shuttleworth, H. "Preventing falls on an elderly care rehabilitation ward", *Clinical Rehabilitation,* 14, pg. 178-185, 2000.

[44] Parker, M. J., Gillespie, L. D., & Gillespie, W. J. "Hip protectors for preventing hip fractures in the elderly", *Cochrane Database of Systematic Reviews,* 1, 2004.

[45] Kannus, P., Parkkari, J., Niemi, S., Pasanen, M., Palvanen, M., Jarvinen, M., et al. "Prevention of hip fracture in elderly people with use of a hip protector", *New England Journal of Medicine,* 343, 1506-1513, 2000.

[46] Cameron, I. D., Venman, J., Kurrle, S. E., Lockwood, K., Birks, C., Cumming, R. G., et al. "Hip protectors in aged-care facilities: a randomized trial of use by individual higher-risk residents", *Age & Ageing,* 30, pgs. 477-81, 2001.

[47] Chan, D. K., Hillier, G., & Coore, M., et al. "Effectiveness and acceptability of a newly designed hip protector: a pilot study", *Archives of Gerontological Geriatrics*, 30, 25-34, 2000.

[48] See note 46.

[49] See note 41.

[50] Talerico, K. A., & Capezuti, E. "Myths and facts about side rails", *American Journal of Nursing*, 101(7), pgs. 43-48, 2001.

[51] Id.

Physical Restraints and Side Rails
by Elizabeth Capezuti

CHAPTER 5

Chapter 5 Physical Restraints and Side Rails
Elizabeth Capezuti PhD, RN, FAAN

A. Introduction
Until the late 1980s, restraints were viewed as an intervention to prevent fall-related incidents and injuries. In the last decade, however, physical restraints have been included in the risk analysis of falls and injuries. [1,2] In response to the overwhelming magnitude of restraint use among institutionalized elders and growing empirical evidence that use of physical restraints produces more problems than it solves, the Nursing Home Reform Act (Omnibus Budget Reconciliation Act [OBRA], 1987) was passed in 1987 as a mechanism to reduce, if not eliminate, the use of physical restraint in nursing homes. [3]

After the Omnibus Budget Reconciliation Act implemented in October 1990, and based on MDS quality indicators, physical restraint use has declined by 38 percent. [4] Hospitals and nursing homes have changed their practices.

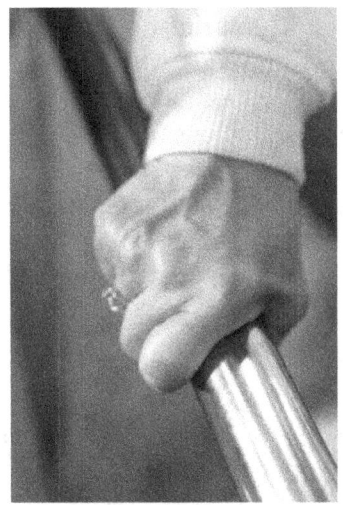

Figure 5-1 Side rails are the source of many injuries

B. Definition
The discussion of restraints and side rails is set within the context of nursing homes, but much of this information is applicable to hospitals. The MDS Trigger defines physical restraints as "Any manual method or physical or mechanical device, material, or equipment attached or adjacent to the resident's body that the individual cannot remove easily which restricts freedom of movement or normal access to one's body." Narrower definitions of restraints exist (e.g. that of the Food and Drug Administration), but practice use of CMS' definition is safest, especially since nursing homes rely on federal Medicare and Medicaid monies. [5]

Physical restraints include chest/vest, pelvic, chest/pelvic combination wrist/mitten/ankle, belt restraints as well as geriatric/recliner/wheelchairs with fixed tray or cushion tables or bars.

> "Posey" is the leading manufacturer of physical restraints; many restraints are now referred to by this brand name (although the restraint may be made by another manufacturer).

Vest/chest restraints are made of polyester/cotton material which fits over the upper torso and can be tied to a chair or bed frame. A pelvic restraint fits over the lower torso similar to a "diaper" but with material ties. A wrist or ankle restraint is made of material or synthetic "sheepskin" and includes ties. The mitten fits over the entire hand to prevent the use of the fingers and includes material to fit snugly around the wrist and ties for attaching to chair/bed. Mittens are sometimes used without the ties.

Belts fit around the waist, thighs or upper torso (shoulder harness), and close with Velcro or a self-release buckle similar to a car seat belt. Although it has a self-release mechanism, it can be considered a restraint if the resident is unable to remove it without physical or verbal assistance. This is the case for the majority of people who have dementia. Belts can also have Velcro closures or buckles that are beyond the reach of the resident, and thus require staff assistance for removal. Belt restraints are used in chairs and bed. A restraining or safety bar is a rigid plastic or metal cylinder that is affixed to a chair near the waist.

Combination restraints restrict movement of several body parts. Examples include the combination chest/pelvic restraint or "Houdini suit," shoulder harness/thigh wheelchair belt, and shoulder harness/waist chair belt. Also, physical restraints can be used with chair restraints and side rails.

"Geriatric" or "geri" chairs and some recliners are vinyl-covered chairs in which the upper torso can be tilted back while the legs are elevated. These, as well as wheelchairs, are restraints when a tray or lap table (either laminated or covered with vinyl) is attached to the chair with a locking mechanism or Velcro ties. A cushion table ("lap-buddy" or "lap-hugger") is a semi-rigid cushion that fits around the waist and wraps around the arms of the chair; it is difficult to remove. A sheet rolled and tied tightly around the waist of a resident's geri-chair or wheelchair or a sheet tucked in tightly under a mattress in a bed-bound resident which restricts movement is also a form of restraint. This type of restraint is referred to as a homemade restraint, and can result in injury through constriction of breathing.

Critical thinking point for the legal nurse consultant: Does the facility institute routine assessment of chairs, table tops and other furniture utilized in practice with older adults, checking on their safety and proper function?

Side rails are adjustable metal or rigid plastic bars that attach to the bed. There are a variety of sizes (full, half, and one-quarter length) and shapes. Most nursing homes have two full-length side rails with wide vertical bars while most hospitals have four "half" or "split" rails attached to the bed. Side rails (of any length) with widely spaced vertical bars, or side rails not situated flush with the mattress are not safe. These side rails can lead to rail and in-bed entrapment and have been associated with asphyxiation deaths.[6]

In 1997 and 1999, CMS issued clear instructions to nursing home administrators: side rails are considered restraints if the resident is able to move and is restricted in getting out of bed by side rails. This includes if a resident's bed is placed against the wall on one side and with a full side rail on the other side, thereby prohibiting the resident from getting in and out of bed. Under CMS Interpretive Guidelines, side rails must be evaluated as a restraint when it serves to both enhance mobility for a resident in bed and simultaneously prohibit getting out of bed.[7] Side rails are not considered restraints if a resident is completely immobile or if the resident requests a side rail to assist in moving in bed or for a feeling of security. For example, a resident with a seizure disorder may have used side rails for several years and feels more comfortable when they are raised. This assumes that the resident is able to give consent to use side rails, recognizing the potential risks associated with their usage. Attempts to reduce the restrictiveness of the side rails can still be tried such as changing two full-length side rails to two upper half side rails.

Critical thinking point: Does the facility clearly distinguish in the training manual the various types of side-rails, their uses, and the hazards when used inappropriately? Are there quality assurance checks to assure that staff utilizes side rails appropriately?

Studies of side rail use in nursing homes suggests a high prevalence of side rails used as restraints - as high as 40 percent to 70 percent amongst nursing home residents.[8] Perhaps this is due to regulations restricting physical restraints, where nursing and ancillary staff may be using side rails to replace "traditional" physical restraints. The side rail is meant by staff to remind residents to call for help and deter them from getting out of bed unassisted. Since most residents with whom side rails are used are cognitively impaired, the rails are actually perceived as a barrier or hurdle to get over or around, leading to greater injury. [9] Side rails can act as restraints and much of the literature continues to preclude the use of side rails as a fall-prevention measure and discourages their use. [1] Interestingly, rates of side rail use in Britain are considerably lower than in the United States [11]; the American use of side rails has even been described as "absurd" and "distasteful" in a British medical journal editorial. [12]

Euphemisms for physical restraints include safety device, reminder belt, protective device, treatment enabler, torso support, security suit, and adaptive or positioning aid. These terms are meaningless. They do not change the intended function of the device: to restrict the ability to move freely. [13]

Restrictions of mobility have most often been justified on the basis of perceived benefits in managing falls and other so-called "problematic" behaviors, including treatment interference, wandering, verbal and physical aggression, and agitation. The literature examining staff attitudes toward restraints corroborates many staff may accept these rationales, [14] pointing to the need for staff education as an area of further development in restraint reduction. With continued restraint use, a growing number of reports of restraint-related injuries and deaths have been a major impetus for reexamining the use of restraints.

Critical thinking point: If occurrences of injury and fatality are documented from restraint use, through a root cause analysis approach did the facility institute any remediation or correction to avoid similar incidents from occurring?

C. Restraint/Side Rail-Related Injuries, Including Death

Neither physical restraints nor side rails have ever been shown to reduce falls or associated injury. [15][16][17] In fact, in the last twenty years there have been numerous reports of restraint-related injuries reported in the professional literature, by the Food and Drug Administration (FDA) and the Joint Commission. Many of these injuries are due to attempts to remove restraints or to ambulate while restrained. These include neurological injuries [18][19] stress-induced complications related to agitation secondary to restraint, [20] and strangulation. [21][22] The most common mechanism of restraint-related death is by asphyxiation; the person is suspended by a restraint from a bed/chair and the ability to inhale is inhibited by gravitational chest compression [23][24] For example in *Estate of Hendrickson v. Genesis Health Ventures, Inc.*, 151 N.C. App. 139, 565 S.E.2d 254 (2002), a plaintiff verdict resulted after a resident died of positional asphyxiation when her head was caught between the mattress and side rail. The same factual scenario also resulted in a plaintiff's verdict in *Bryant v. Oakpointe Villa Nursing Centre*, 2004 MICH. LEXIS 1699.

There is a growing amount of forensic medicine literature describing the medical examiner's role in evaluating these cases of restraint-related death. As there are often no eye witnesses at the time of death, an effort is made to piece together available evidence. In many cases, classic signs of asphyxia such as neck bruising may be absent and atypical compression of the neck by bedrails may be the cause of death (i.e. the respiratory tract was compressed without damaging the subcutaneous tissues, cartilage, or bone). [25]

In response to the increasing number of reports of these injuries, many organizations have issued statements or guidelines discouraging the use of physical restraints. The FDA issued regulations requiring that healthcare facilities report serious injuries to the manufacturer and restraint-related deaths to both the

FDA and manufacturer.[26] After receiving numerous reports of injuries and deaths, the FDA in September of 1992 proposed for the first time that manufacturers be required to provide results of safety and effectiveness studies of physical restraints.[27] Similarly, the FDA issued a Safety Alert in 1995 concerning hazards associated with the use of side rails. The Alert described sixty-eight deaths and twenty-two injuries associated with 102 reports of head and body entrapment incidents involving side rails.[28]

Since April 1999, the FDA in conjunction with representatives from the hospital bed industry, healthcare organizations, patient advocacy groups, and other government agencies convened the Hospital Bed Safety Workgroup. Its goal is to improve the safety of hospital beds in all healthcare settings to prevent injury and protect vulnerable patients at risk of entrapment. The Workgroup developed guidelines and educational materials for caregivers and consumers, focusing on individualized assessment and restraint reduction.[29] On August 30, 2004, draft guidelines regarding the dimensions of hospital beds and their accessories (e.g., side rail) were published in the *Federal Register*.[30]

All accredited healthcare organizations must report serious adverse events to the Joint Commission. These sentinel events are studied to identify causes, trends, and outcomes in order to provide important information to prevent future sentinel events. Joint Commission noted that as many as 8 percent of sentinel events in healthcare facilities were restraint-related deaths in 1998 and 2001. These alarming statistics led Joint Commission to issue Sentinel Event Alerts including risk reduction strategies such as equipment redesign to reduce gaps and openings for entrapment. Key recommendations also involve educating staff and the resident/family about the purpose and dangers of bed rails. Recent Joint Commission data shows a reduction of restraint deaths to 4 percent of sentinel events.[31]

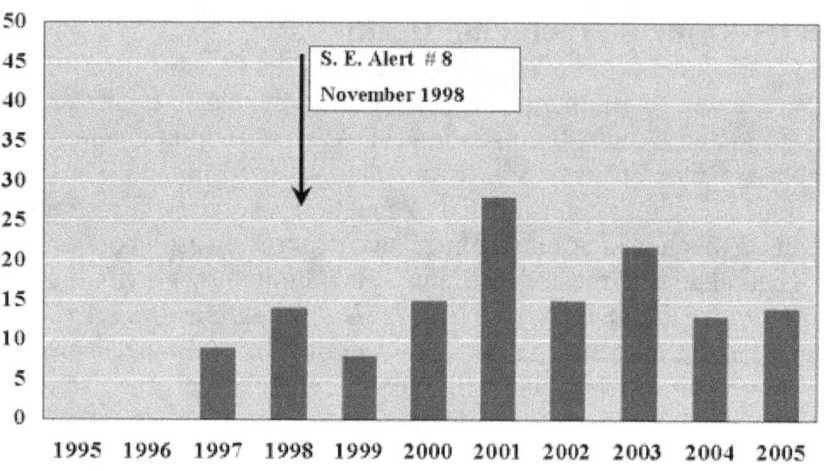

Figure 5-2 http://www.jointcommission.org/NR/rdonlyres/819F7EBE-8AD7-432B-8493-DBAC4956B54D/0/se_trends_restraint_events.gif

> *Critical thinking point for clinicians:* Through review of incident report analysis and monthly tabulations, can you determine if sentinel events related to restraint use-fatality are increasing, decreasing, or remaining the same?

In addition to the FDA and Joint Commission, as mentioned, AGS [32] and AMDA [33] have position statements advocating the reduction of all types of restraint use. Obviously, physical restraint, including side rail use, is not a benign treatment; it does have serious risks. Aside from physical injury, restraint application may also result in significant psychological damage including depression, fear, and humiliation, further decreasing a resident's quality of life. [34]

Those healthcare providers that choose to ignore FDA alerts regarding patient injuries do so at their own peril. In Texas, a July 2003 case described below resulted in a verdict of $2,975,000.00 for a positional asphyxiation death due to side rail entrapment. Part of the jury's focus in this case was the fact that defendants ignored a prior FDA alert.

> Consider the *Charles v. Baptist Hospital of Southwest Texas, et al* of Jefferson County Texas District Court Case E-163355. Morris Charles, age seventy, was admitted to Baptist Hospital for symptoms which were later discovered to have been caused by a subdural hematoma from a fall he had a few weeks prior to this treatment. During his admissions, he was restrained without signed orders from the doctors. On September 3, 1998, he was restrained with bilateral wrist restraints and side rails. He was found by a nurse's aide with the lower half of his body through the gap between the upper and lower side rail, and his neck and upper chest wedged between the side rail and the air mattress. Discovery from the bed manufacturer showed that it was aware of the risk of patient entrapment from reports received from health care providers that it investigated. The FDA issued an alert to biomedical engineers and healthcare providers indicating that elderly confused patients were a high risk, and there had been deaths reported. KCI regulatory affairs director received the FDA alert, but did not forward it to his engineering staff, or to his customer service staff. The Estate of Morris Charles was awarded $625,000 for physical pain and mental anguish before death. Veronica Charles was awarded $550,000 loss of companionship in the past, $500,000 future loss of companionship, $650,000 past mental anguish, and $650,000 future mental anguish—for a total for Veronica of $2,350,000. The total jury award was $2,975,000. [35]

D. Recent Research/Clinical Practice Regarding the Relationship to Falls/Injuries

Unfortunately, some "common" practices, such as restraint use prior to OBRA '87, were attributed to "common sense". [36] Numerous studies, however, have described a significant incidence of falls and serious injury in restrained elders. [37][38][39][40] The studies provide empirical evidence for the ineffectiveness of restraints in fall prevention.

> The dramatic decrease in restraint use post-OBRA has not resulted in significant increases in injurious falls.

Several carefully conducted studies of the effect of restraint reduction have demonstrated no increase in falls or injurious falls. [41][42][43][44][45][46][47] Further, there has never been a published scientific report demonstrating the efficacy of side rails in preventing falls and resulting injuries from bed. Their usage, similar to physical restraints, is based on a "common-sense" notion of preventing falls from bed. [48][49][50]

Since side rails create physical barriers for residents getting out of bed, they often increase the height of the fall by two feet. [51] Falls from a standing height or higher are more likely to result in hip fracture. [52] Recently reported studies demonstrated that residents in bed without side rails were no more likely to fall from bed than those with side rails. [53][54][55]

Regulations discouraging the use of physical restraints (including side rails) and warnings from the FDA and research demonstrating the risk of harmful and even fatal effects verify that restraints are neither safe nor effective devices for fall prevention. Professional standards restricting their use must be considered in both a fall case and a restraint-related injury/death case. [56][57][58][59]

E. Standards Related to Use of Physical Restraints

Physical restraints, including side rails, can only be used after obtaining informed consent from the resident, or if the resident is decisionally incapable, the resident's surrogate decision maker. With informed consent, the resident and family are included in the decision-making process. The physician is responsible for discussing the risks of restraint/side rail use, including injury and death, as recommended by the American Medical Association's Council on Scientific Affairs, [60] as well as according to CMS regulations.

Critical thinking point for clinicians: Instead of believing that failure to use restraints puts you at risk for legal liability, are you aware that lack of assessment and care planning to address fall risk is the greatest hazard? Physical restraint is no longer viewed by professionals or governmental agencies overseeing nursing homes as a treatment to prevent falls. Successful cases for plaintiff should be based on facts demonstrating that staff that did not appropriately address the patient's risk of falling.

Prior to OBRA '87, physical restraints were considered common sense interventions and did not explicitly require a physician's prescription or order. OBRA '87 requires physician orders. Since 1997, CMS has clarified this regulation to include side rails. However, a decisionally-capable resident can refuse a physician's order for restraint. For example, a plaintiff alleged that a fractured hip secondary to a fall from bed was due to a failure to use two full-length side rails. The defense contended that the resident refused two side rails, resulting in a defense verdict. [61] Nursing homes are also regulated by state law, such as Colorado law which limits physical restraint use to emergency situations and when no less restrictive alternative is possible. [62] Use of physical restraint must also demonstrate a process of professional judgment. [63] Since 1997, side rails used as restraints also require the same individualized assessment and plan of care as physical restraints. [64] The decision to use restraint is not limited to the physician. Professional judgment must also be demonstrated by a multidisciplinary assessment and plan of care (usually documented in the interdisciplinary care plan and/or a specific restraint/fall assessment form specific to the facility). Restraint use (physical and side rails) must be documented in the MDS and the RAPS including trials of alternative interventions toward reducing restraint use (as described in the intervention section). Tag number F221 in the surveyor's manual details definitions of restraints and instances in which their use is prohibited. [65]

Each facility must have a policy and procedure that includes the decision-making process of physical restraint use. This process includes evaluation of all members of the multidisciplinary clinical team (nurse, physician, social worker and physical and occupational therapist).

Family members or other resident surrogate decision makers cannot request that a restraint be used on a resident without the multidisciplinary clinical team's endorsement. They do not have "the right to demand potentially hazardous treatments that do not have a therapeutic benefit". [66] In all instances, restraints may never be used for the sake of discipline, staff convenience, or when restraints are not necessary to treat the resident's medical symptoms. The nursing home is compelled to provide care that is in the best interest of the resident. It is well recognized that most decision-making regarding restraints are made by nurses. [67][68][69] The vast majority of nursing home physicians are off-site in private practice and visit their patient and renew orders monthly. [70] Thus, day-to-day monitoring is done by nurses (most often, licensed practical/vocational nurses) who are responsible to inform the physician of changes in the resident's condition (e.g. falls) and suggest treatment orders (e.g. medication changes, physical therapy consultation, etc.). This communication is usually conducted over the telephone and changes in orders are written by the nurse as "telephone verbal orders". [71] Thus, nurses have a great deal of influence for orders, including restraints. [72] Researchers have developed nursing guidelines for individualized assessment and interventions with side rail use. [73] Tools to guide side rail usage include the *Side Rail and Alternative Equipment Intervention Decision Tree,* [74] and the *Evaluation of Side Rail Usage* questionnaire, an individualized assessment tool for use by a restraint reduction committee. [75]

The OBRA '87 regulations are meant to reduce restraint orders without multidisciplinary evaluation and a trial of non-restraint interventions. A restraint order must be preceded (unless the person is an *immediate*, life-threatening danger to self or others) by a documented evaluation. The physician's order must be renewed at least monthly. The multidisciplinary team must reevaluate its use at least quarterly or if there is a change of condition related to the restraint (e.g. resident is found hanging from the bed while continuing to be tied down with a restraint).

> The nursing staff is required to document release of the restraint, followed by exercise (minimally, range of motion of the restrained joint) and toileting (or change of adult incontinence pad or "diaper") for ten minutes every two hours. One study found that staff rarely adhered to this directive. [76]

A study examining costs noted that such care during restraint use would require increased staff levels. [77] These regulations are meant to combat the sequelae of prolonged restraint use: deconditioning, pressure ulcers, contractures, anorexia, decreased mental status, and agitation.

The continued use of restraints including evidence of serious outcomes such as fatality and the appearance (from some limited research studies) that certain required protocols for their use are insufficiently adhered to, serves as a catalyst for the new CMS regulations. Regulations from CMS call for better and more extensive training of healthcare workers who employ physical restraints and seclusion when treating patients, in order to assure the appropriateness of the treatment and to protect patient rights as cited in the *Federal Register*. "The patients' rights regulations set forth, as a condition of participation (CoP) in the Medicare and Medicaid programs, the expectation that health care facilities will protect the rights of patients." All participating hospitals including short-term, psychiatric, rehabilitation, long-term, children's and alcohol/drug treatment facilities are affected. According to the acting director of the CMS, this regulation reinforces "this administration's commitment to patient safety and the delivery of high quality healthcare services." [78]

The outcome of this regulation will spur the development and implementation of quality improvement training programs that uniformly send the same message to be followed. Healthcare outcomes to be realized as a spin off from this regulation include improved patient care, and lessened incidences of geriatric syndromes associated with deconditioning, disuse, immobility, agitation, pressure sores and other preventable events. The evidence shows that physical restraints and side rails as interventions for the prevention of falls either do not work or create additional problems such as morbidity and fatality. In any event, their use is becoming increasingly hazardous and obsolete, except in the cases of emergency protocol which may justify some limited use. Providers should replace the physical restraint, in clinically indicated situations, with interventions which have some basis of effectiveness in reducing agitation or preventing falls. A wealth of nursing interventions are available for this very purpose and must be utilized when following the nursing process. Failure to do so creates negligent care and can spur litigation. The next chapter addresses the legal process related to the standard of care for fall prevention.

End notes

[1] Rawnsky, E. "Review of the literature on falls among the elderly", *Image: Journal of Nursing Scholarship*, 30, pgs. 47-52, 1998.

[2] Capezuti, E., Evans, L., Strumpf, N., et al. "Physical restraint use and falls in nursing home residents", *Journal of the American Geriatrics Society,* 44, pgs. 627-633, 1996.

[3] Contained within the Omnibus Budget Reconciliation Act of 1987 (OBRA-87, 42 Omnibus Budget Reconciliation Act of 1987, Public Law No. 100-203, Title IV, subtitle C, sections 4201-4206, 4211-4216, 101 Stat 1330-160 through 1330-220, 42 USC section 1395; -3(a)-(h) {Medicaid}(1992). U.S.C. §§ 1395i & 1396 *et seq;* [83])

[4] Centers for Medicare and Medicaid. Nursing Home Compare website. [Online] Retrieved March 31, 2006 from Internet at: http://www.medicare.gov/NHCompare/Include/DataSection/Questions/SearchCriteria.asp?version=default&browser=IE%7C6%7CwinXP&language=English&defaultstatus=0&pagelist=Home&CookiesEnabledStatus=True.

[5] Talerico, K. A., & Capezuti, E. "Myths and facts about side rails", *American Journal of Nursing*, 101(7), pgs. 43-48, 2001.

[6] Parker, K., & Miles, S. H. "Deaths caused by bedrails", *Journal of the American Geriatrics Society,* 45, pgs. 797-802, 1997.

[7] Capezuti, E. A., & Braun, J. A. "Medico-legal aspects of hospital side rail use", *Ethics, Law, and Aging Review*, 7, pgs. 25-57, 2001.

[8] Capezuti, E., Maislin, G., Strumpf, N., & Evans, L. K. "Side rail use and bed-related fall outcomes among nursing home residents", *Journal of the American Geriatrics Society,* 50, pgs.90-96, 2002.

[9] Capezuti, E. "Preventing falls and injuries while reducing side rail use", *Annals of Long-Term Care*, 8(6), pgs. 57-63, 2000. Also available: http://www.nursing.upenn.edu/centers/hcgne/

[10] See note 8.

[11] O'Keefe, S., Jack, C. I., & Lye, M. "Use of restraints and bedrails in a British hospital", *Journal of the American Geriatrics Society,* 44, pgs. 1086-1088, 1996.

[12] Anonymous. "Cotsides: protecting whom against what?" *Lancet,* 35, pg. 383-384, 1984.

[13] See note 3.

[14] Hardin, S. B., Magee, R., Stratmann, D., Vinson, M. H., Owen, M., & Hyatt, E. C. "Extended care and nursing home staff attitudes toward restraints", *Journal of Gerontological Nursing,* 20, pg. 23-31, 1994.

[15] American Geriatrics Society, British Geriatrics Society, American Academy of Orthopedic Surgeons Panel on Falls Prevention. "Guidelines for the prevention of falls in older persons", *Journal of the American Geriatrics Society,* 49(5), pgs. 664-681, 2001.

[16] Ray, W. A., Taylor, J. A., Meador, K. G., Thapa, P. B., Brown, A. K., Kajihara, H. K., et al. "A randomized trial of a consultation service to reduce falls in nursing homes", *Journal of the American Medical Association,* 278, pgs. 557-562, 1997.

[17] Agency for Health Care Policy and Research. Making Health Care Safer: A Critical Analysis of Patient Safety Practices. File Inventory, Evidence Report/Technology Assessment Number 43. AHRQ Publication No. 01-E058, Rockville, MD. 2001. Chapter 26: Prevention of Falls in Hospitalized and Institutionalized Older People, J. Agostini, D. Baker, S. Bogardus (Authors). Retrieved May 15, 2004 from http://www.ahrq.gov/clinic/ptsftinv.htm

[18] Skeen, M. B., Rozear, M. P., & Morgenlander, J. C. "Posey palsy", *Annals of Internal Medicine,* 117 (9), pg. 795, 1992.

[19] Vogel, C. M., & Bromberg, M. B. "Proximal upper extremity compressive neuropathy associated with prolonged use of a jacket restraint", {Abstract}. *Muscle Nerve*, 13, pg. 860, 1990.

[20] Robinson, B. E., Sucholeiki, R., & Schocken, D.D. "Sudden death and resisted mechanical restraint: a case report", *Journal of the American Geriatrics Society*, 41, pgs.424-425, 1993.

[21] DiMaio, V.J.M., Dana, S. E., & Bux, R. C. "Deaths caused by vest restraint", *Journal of the American Medical Association,* 255, pg. 905, 1986.

[22] Dube, A. H., & Mitchell, E. K. "Accidental strangulation from vest restraints", *Journal of the American Medical Association,* 256, pgs. 2725-2726.S, 1986

[23] DiNunno, N., Vacca, M., Costantinedes, F., & DiNunno, C. "Death following atypical compression of the neck", *American Journal of Forensic Medicine and Pathology*, 24, pgs.364-368, 2003.

[24] Miles, S. H. "Deaths between bedrails and air pressure mattresses", *Journal of the American Geriatrics Society,* 50, pgs. 1124-1125, 2002.

[25] See note 23.

[26] Weick, M. D. "Physical restraints: An FDA update", *American Journal of Nursing,* 92 (11), pgs. 74-80, 1992.

[27] "New Regulatory Controls for Patient Restraints from FDA Medical Bulletin", *Untie the Elderly*, 4 (3), 3. September, 1992.

[28] Burlington, D. B. *Entrapment hazards with hospital bed side rails. FDA Safety Alert.* Rockville, MD: Food and Drug Administration, Public Health Service, Department of Health and Human Services, August 23, 1995.

[29] Hospital Bed Safety Workgroup, "Clinical guidance for the assessment and implementation of bed rails in hospital, long term care facilities, and home care settings", Available on Internet at http://www.fda.gov/cdrh/beds/. (2003, April).

[30] See note 23.

[31] Reason, J. *Human Error*: New York: Cambridge University Press, 1990.

[32] American Geriatrics Society, British Geriatrics Society, American Academy of Orthopedic Surgeons Panel on Falls Prevention. "Guidelines for the prevention of falls in older persons", *Journal of the American Geriatrics Society,* 49(5), pgs. 664-681, 2001.

[33] American Medical Directors Association (AMDA) and The American Health Care Association (1998; 2003) *Falls and Fall Risk: Clinical Practice Guideline,* American Medical Directors Association, Columbia, MD. [Online]. Available on Internet at: http://www.amda.com/clinical/falls/figure_1.htm

[34] Guttman, R., Altman, R. D., & Karlan, M. S. "Report of the Council on Scientific Affairs: use of restraints for patients in nursing homes", *Archives of Family Medicine*, 8, pgs.101-105, 1999.

[35] Laska, L. (Ed). *Charles v. Baptist Hospital of Southwest Texas, et al* Jefferson County Texas District, *Medical Malpractice Verdicts, Settlements, and Experts*, July, 2003.

[36] Rubenstein, H. S., Miller, F. H., Postel, S., et al. "Standards of medical care based on consensus rather than evidence: The case of routine bedrail use for the elderly", *Law, Medicine and Health Care,* 11, pgs. 271-276, 1983.

[37] Hawes, C., Mor, V., Phillips, C.D., Fries, B.E., Morris, J.N., Steele-Friedlob, E., Greene, A.M., Nennstiel, M. "The OBRA-87 nursing home regulations and implementation of the Residents Assessment Instrument: effects on process quality", *Journal of the American Geriatrics Society*, 45 (8), pgs. 977-985, 1997.

[38] Misener, M. & Matteson, M. A. "Fall-related injury in nursing home residents", {Abstract}. *The Gerontologist,* 33 (Special Issue 1), p. 276, 1993.

[39] Neufeld, R. R., Libow, L. S., Foley, W. J., Dunbar, J. M., Cohen, C., & Breuer, B. "Restraint reduction reduces serious injuries among nursing home residents", *Journal of the American Geriatrics Society, 47,* pgs.1202-1207, 1999.

[40] Tinetti, M. E., Liu, W. L., & Ginter, S. F. "Mechanical restraint use and fall-related injuries among residents of skilled nursing facilities", *Annals of Internal Medicine,* 116, pgs. 369-374, 1992

[41] Cali, C. M., & Kiel, D. P. "An epidemiologic study of fall-related fractures among institutionalized older people", *Journal of the American Geriatrics Society,* 43, pgs. 1336-1340, 1995.

[42] Capezuti, E., Strumpf, N., Evans, L., et al. "The relationship between physical restraint removal and falls and injuries among nursing home residents", *Journal of Gerontology: Medical Sciences, 53A,* pgs. M47-M53, 1998.

[43] Ejaz, F. K., Jones, J. A., & Rose, M. S. "Falls among nursing home residents: an examination of incident reports before and after restraint reduction programs", *Journal of the American Geriatrics Society,* 42, pgs. 960-964, 1994.

[44] Evans, L. K., Strumpf, N. E., Allen-Taylor, S. L., et al. "A clinical trial to reduce restraints in nursing homes", *Journal of the American Geriatrics Society,* 45, pgs. 675-681, 1997.

[45] Kramer, J.D. (1994). "educing restraint used in a nursing home", *Clinical Nurse Specialist,* 8, pgs. 158-162, 1994.

[46] Stratmann, D., Vinson, M. H., Magee et al. (1997). "The effects of research on clinical practice: The use of restraints", *Applied Nursing Research*, 10, pgs. 39-43, 1997.

[47] Werner, P., Cohen-Mansfield, J., Koroknay, V., et al. "The impact of a restraint-reduction program on nursing home residents", *Geriatric Nursing,* 15, pgs.142-146, 1994.

[48] See note 8.

[49] Id.

[50] Agency for Health Care Policy and Research. Making Health Care Safer: A Critical Analysis of Patient Safety Practices. File Inventory, Evidence Report/Technology Assessment Number 43. AHRQ Publication No. 01-E058, Rockville, MD. 2001. Chapter 26: Prevention of Falls in Hospitalized and Institutionalized Older People, J. Agostini, D. Baker, S. Bogardus (Authors). Retrieved May 15, 2004 from http://www.ahrq.gov/clinic/ptsftinv.htm

[51] Grisso, J. A., Capezuti, E., & Schwartz, A. "Falls as risk factors for fractures", In R. Arcus, D. Feldman and J. Kelsey (Eds.). *Osteoporosis.* San Diego: Academic Press, 1996.

[52] Grisso, J. A., Kelsey, J. L., Strom, B. L., et al. "Risk factors for falls as a cause of hip fracture in women", *New England Journal of Medicine,* 324, pgs.1326-1330, 1991.

[53] Hanger, H. C., Ball, M. C., & Wood, L. A. "An analysis of falls in the hospital: can we do without bedrails?" *Journal of the American Geriatrics Society,* 47, pgs. 529-531, 1999.

[54] Si, M., Neufeld, R. R., & Dunbar, J. "Removal of bedrails on a short-term nursing home rehabilitation unit", *Gerontologist,* 39, pgs. 611-614, 1999.

[55] Hanger, H. C., Ball, M. C., & Wood, L. A. "An analysis of falls in the hospital: can we do without bedrails?" *Journal of the American Geriatrics Society,* 47, pgs. 529-531, 1999.

[56] Capezuti, E. A. Falls. In M.A. Forciea and R. Lavizzo-Mourey (Eds.) *Geriatric Secrets*. Philadelphia: Hanley and Belfus, 1996.

[57] Johnson, R., and Beneda, H. "Reducing patient restraint use*",* *Nursing Management,* 29, pgs. 32-34, 1998.

[58] Strumpf, N. E., Robinson, J. P., Wagner, J. S., et al. *Restraint-free Care.* New York: Springer, 1998.

[59] Stratmann, D., Vinson, M. H., Magee et al. (1997). "The effects of research on clinical practice: The use of restraints", *Applied Nursing Research*, 10, pgs. 39-43, 1997.

[60] Guttman, R., Altman, R. D., & Karlan, M. S. "Report of the Council on Scientific Affairs: use of restraints for patients in nursing homes", *Archives of Family Medicine, 8*, pgs.101-105, 1999.

[61] Laska, L. (Ed). "Failure to properly restrain patient", *Medical Malpractice Verdicts, Settlements and Experts,* pg. 27, December, 1997.

[62] Tinetti, M. E., Liu, W. L., & Ginter, S. F. "Mechanical restraint use and fall-related injuries among residents of skilled nursing facilities", *Annals of Internal Medicine,* 116, pgs. 369-374, 1992.

[63] Cohen, E. S., and Kruschwitz, A. L. "Restraint reduction: Lessons from the asylum", *Ethics, Law, and Aging,* 3, pgs. 25-43, 1997.

[64] Johnson, R., and Beneda, H. "Reducing patient restraint use*", Nursing Management,* 29, pgs. 32-34, 1998.

[65] Hardin, S. B., Magee, R., Stratmann, D., Vinson, M. H., Owen, M., & Hyatt, E. C. "Extended care and nursing home staff attitudes toward restraints", *Journal of Gerontological Nursing,* 20, pg. 23-31, 1994.

[66] Miles, S. "Looking at bedrail and vest deaths: perspectives of an expert witness", *Untie the Elderly*, 10, pgs.1-3, 1998.

[67] Cohen-Mansfield, J., Marx, M. S., & Werner, P. "Restraining cognitively impaired nursing home residents", *Nursing Management,* 24, pgs. 112Q-112W, 1993.

[68] Phillips, C. D., Hawes, C., Mor, V., et al. "Facility and area variation affecting the use of physical restraints in nursing homes", *Medical Care,* 34, pgs.1149-1162, 1996.

[69] Schnelle, J. F., Simmons, S. F., & Ory, M. G. (1992). "Risk factors that predict staff failure to release nursing home residents from restraints", *The Gerontologist,* 32, pgs.767-770, 1992.

[70] Capezuti, E., & Siegler, E. L. "The role of the academic nurse and physician in the criminal prosecution of nursing home mistreatment" *Journal of Elder Abuse and Neglect,* 8, pgs. 47-58, 1996.

[71] Id

[72] Kayser-Jones, J. "Decision making in the treatment of acute illness in nursing homes: Framing the decision problem, treatment plan, and outcome", *Medical Anthropology Quarterly*, 9, pgs. 236-256, 1995.

[73] Capezuti, E., Talerico, K. A., Cochran, I., Becker, H., Strumpf, N., & Evans, L. "Individualized interventions to reduce falls from bed and bilateral side rail use", *Journal of Gerontological Nursing,* 25, pgs. 26-34, 1999.

[74] Talerico, K. A., & Capezuti, E. "Myths and facts about side rails", *American Journal of Nursing*, 101(7), pgs. 43-48, 2001.

[75] Capezuti, E. "Preventing falls and injuries while reducing side rail use", *Annals of Long-Term Care*, 8(6), pgs. 57-63, 2000. Also available: http://www.nursing.upenn.edu/centers/hcgne/

[76] Schnelle, J. F., Simmons, S. F., & Ory, M. G. "Risk factors that predict staff failure to release nursing home residents from restraints", *The Gerontologist,* 32, pgs.767-770, 1992

[77] Phillips, C. D., Hawes, C., & Fries, B. E. "Reducing the use of physical restraints in nursing homes: Will it increase costs", *American Journal of Public Health*, 83, pgs.342-346, 1993

[78] http://frwebgate2.access.gpo.gov/cgi-bin/waisgate.cgi?WAISdocID=835580397202+0+0+0&WAISaction=retrieve. http://www.cms.hhs.gov/apps/media/press/release.asp?Counter=2057&intNumPerPage=10&checkDate=&checkKey=&srchType=&numDays=3500&srchOpt=0&srchData=&keywordType=All&chkNewsType=1%2C+2%2C+3%2C+4%2C+5&intPage=&showAll=&pYear=&year=&desc=false&cboOrder=date

Legal Aspects of Falls
by Elizabeth Capezuti
William Lawson
Patricia Iyer

CHAPTER 6

Chapter 6 Legal Aspects of Falls
Elizabeth Capezuti, PhD, RN, FAAN, William T. Lawson, III, JD, and Patricia Iyer MSN RN LNCC

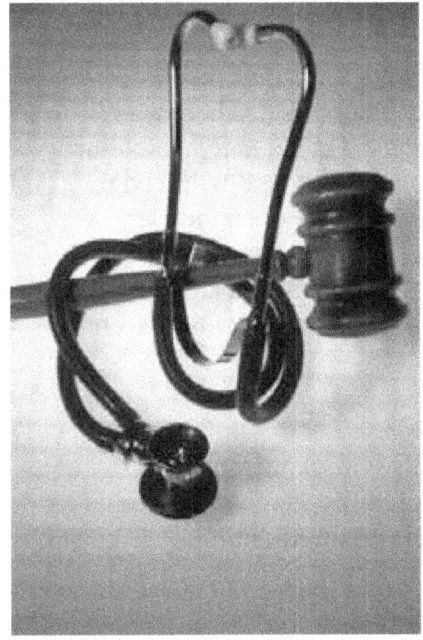

Figure 6-1 The intersection of law and medicine

A. The Legal Process

Falls are the most common reason nurses or their healthcare employers are sued. The legal process usually begins with a phone call to a plaintiff's attorney reporting facts consistent with a fall. The person at the firm receiving the call (attorney, legal nurse consultant, paralegal, secretary) will ask the caller a number of questions:

- What kind of injury occurred as a result of the fall?
- What is the condition of the person now?
- What is your relationship to the person who was injured?
- (This is asked to determine if this person has the legal
- authority to act on behalf of the injured person.)
- What do you think was done wrong?
- Did anyone admit that something was done wrong?
- Where did the fall occur?
- When did the fall occur?

1. Damages/injuries

The information gathered in this call will determine if it is worthwhile arranging an appointment for the caller to meet with the attorney. Before committing to prosecute a fall case, the law firm personnel carefully examine damages issues. While callers may describe one or even many falls which are potentially valid claims, a large portion of the decision making process centers upon the damages or injuries. Attorneys are most likely to pursue cases where the injury results in a permanent negative impact on the patient's activities of daily living. [1] Fractured hips, head injuries leading to subdural or subarachnoid hemorrhages, paralysis from spinal cord injuries, and death are significant damages.

2. Caller's relationship to patient

As simple as it may initially seem, the process of determining who the plaintiffs are can be quite vexing. Just as difficult is the issue involving which individuals might have standing to assert claims on behalf of injured parties. When the injured party is a minor, parents generally can and will serve as Guardian ad Litem. There are occasions, though, when the Court may want or need to appoint an independent Guardian – typically an attorney. This can occur when a conflict of interest arises or when the judgment of the parents appears to be antithetical to the interests of the child. When the injured party is a mentally competent adult, the assessment is much simpler. However, claims recorded during the intake phase of a case are anything but simple when divorce or separation occurs during a malpractice suit. [2]

3. Caller's perceptions of what was done wrong

The evolving standard of care related to restraints and side rail use is not universally known by all healthcare providers, much less the public. The caller may say, "I told them to tie down my mother. I knew she would get out of bed." This claim would be explored to determine what fall prevention measures were put into place in lieu of using restraints. On the other hand, the caller may say, "I told them they needed to watch her. She needed to be in a ground floor room in the nursing home. Instead, they put her on the second floor. She fell going down the stairs." See Case Three in the Appendix. This case reflects a different level of liability and would more likely be investigated by the attorney.

4. Admissions and apologies

There is increasing awareness that it is important to talk with families and patients after an incident resulting in injury has occurred. The timing and nature of the disclosure of information during this conversation is the subject of much debate. The Joint Commission published a standard in 2001 that required healthcare providers to inform patients and their families about unanticipated outcomes. An immediate outcry was heard from risk managers, doctors, and others who were fearful of the implications of telling patients the truth about errors. Compliance with this standard is not universal. There is still considerable resistance and fear rooted in the perception that admitting mistakes is not safe in a culture that still subscribes to blame and punishment as methods for ensuring accountability and will lead to litigation. [3] Many people contact law firms after injuries occurred because they have been unable to get appropriate answers from the healthcare providers involved in the incident. Several states have passed laws that permit apologies to be given to patients without it being used against the healthcare providers. A person residing in a state with an apology a law is not prevented for pursuing a claim, however. Refer to www.sorryworks.net for more information.

5. Location of the fall

The location and nature of the facility where the fall took place is also of great significance. Legal restrictions may be placed on the attorney's ability to file a claim against a facility that has charitable immunity. Most states have some type of statute rendering such facilities either totally immune from suit or limiting damages. When such an institution is named in a lawsuit, attorneys will frequently identify nurses who provided care to the individual. This can often result in some amount of legal friction between the nurse and his or her employing institution or place of contractual engagement. Many more hospitals than nursing homes will be subject to the local jurisdiction's charitable immunity statute simply by virtue of the means by which many hospitals are established and taxed. [4] Other restrictions on claims are affected by minimal or lack of insurance coverage.

6. Date of the fall

The statute of limitations also affects the viability of a claim. For example, a state with a two year statute of limitation will generally require that a complaint be filed no later than two years from the time of the injury. [5] In limited cases this period may be extended by the discovery rule or if the facility fraudulently conceals information. In many cases, the statute of limitations will be extended when the injured person is mentally incompetent. While it is certainly preferable to avoid all of these issues from the plaintiff's point of view and simply file suit within the appropriate statute of limitations, families frequently do not approach counsel in sufficient time to meet all of these statutes of limitations. Thus, many claims which appear to have otherwise expired have not when the injured party was mentally incompetent for either all or part of the time that the incidents occurred. [6]

Assuming that the caller has provided information that warrants further investigation, an appointment is set up to have the individual meet the plaintiff's attorney. During this meeting, more information is obtained about the fall. Medical records are obtained and evaluated to determine if the care provided conformed to the standard of care. When evaluating the fall case, the reviewer will consider three factors: the seriousness of the injury, the circumstances surrounding the fall, and the measures the personnel took before and after the fall.

In summary, liability issues that attorneys consider in screening a fall case include:

- How did the fall occur?
- Was the patient appropriately identified as being at risk for falls?

- Was a plan of care implemented to reduce the risk for falls?
- Was the fall/injury promptly reported (versus being concealed)?
- What changes in the plan of care were made to reduce the risk of subsequent falls?
- Were these successful? [7]

B. Standard of Care as a Dynamic Concept

Falls and fall related injuries represent a significant number of lawsuits involving nurses. [8] Basic tort law applies to all professional malpractice cases. In order to maintain an action for professional malpractice, there must be a violation of the prevailing standard of care, which is the proximate cause of an injury, resulting in damages. The deviation from the prevailing standard of care may be by affirmative actions (e.g., leaving an obstacle in the path of a person) or by acts of omission (e.g., not supervising a room full of cognitively impaired patients). Standards are "benchmarks of clinical performance and practice by ... an average qualified practitioner exercising a reasonable degree of care and skill ... taking into account advances in the profession." [9] The standard of care used to evaluate a case, therefore, must be based on the governmental regulations and clinical/professional standards in effect at the time the fall took place. Governmental regulations are based on federal law governing Medicare and Medicaid and state licensing statutes. [10] Professional standards for practice are ideally based on scientific evidence. The federal government, through the Agency for Healthcare Research and Quality (AHRQ), has produced monographs summarizing and evaluating the latest assessment techniques and interventions for many clinical problems, such as pressure ulcers and urinary incontinence. Although there is no established AHRQ guideline for falls, AHRQ describes safety practices to reduce falls and restraint use in their publications; there is also an abundance of medical, nursing, and rehabilitation articles written in professional journals. Each healthcare facility may have its own policy on falls; these policies must reflect current governmental regulations and professional standards.

C. Professional Policies and Guidelines

In addition to federal and state regulation, professional organizations have developed policies and clinical practice guidelines regarding falls prevention and restraint use. For example, the American Geriatrics Society (AGS) produced a position statement advocating the reduction of all types of restraint use and presenting guidelines for their use in the uncommon instances that they are needed. [11] AGS has also, in conjunction with the British Geriatrics Society and the American Academy of Orthopedic Surgeons, developed an evidence-based guideline for falls prevention in older adults. [12]

The USPSTF (U.S. Preventive Services Task Force) recommends that all people 75 years or older, and those 70 to 74 years old with a known risk factor, should be counseled about specific measures to prevent falls. The American Medical Directors Association, composed of medical directors and physicians practicing in long term care, published their own clinical practice guidelines in 1998 (and updated in 2003) on falls and fall risk. [13] The aim of the guidelines is to assist practitioners to identify ways to modify some risk factors for falls, as well as ways to adjust the patient's environment to minimize the risk of injury due to falls. Similar to the USPSTF guideline, this guideline supports multifactorial interventions in long-term care, including staff education programs, gait training, and advice on assistive device use, and review and adjustment of medications, especially psychoactive medications. Screening measures are an important component of these guidelines. The AGS guideline does not stipulate an age at which screening should begin, but recommends that all elderly patients be asked about any falls that have occurred during the past year and should undergo a quick test of gait and balance. The "get up and go" test is performed by asking the person to get up from a chair, walk a few feet, turn, and sit down.

Critical thinking point for clinicians: Do you apply your clinical knowledge and use your professional judgment in following the fall prevention recommendations? There is always an element of subjectivity in practice. Implementation of clinical practice guidelines should be evaluated and facilitate the development of falls prevention programs. [14] Nevertheless, policy statements and guidelines set forth by major organizations are often held by the courts to be appropriate standards of care and may be considered as evidence of the standard of care.

D. Common Allegations in Fall Cases

A review of 253 nursing malpractice claims dealing with many different types of claims revealed that the allegations fit into one of these six categories:
- failure to follow standards of care;
- failure to use equipment in a responsible manner;
- failure to communicate;
- failure to document;
- failure to assess and monitor; and
- failure to act as a patient advocate. [15]

These six allegations apply to fall cases. The plaintiff's expert witness (a person with particular expertise to form opinions about the standard of care) may allege any of these deviations occurred. Below are some examples of deviations alleged in actual fall related cases.

Failure to follow standards of care
- failure to follow the care plan intervention that two people were needed to transfer a patient
- failure to support a paraplegic patient during a shower caused a fall and fractured pelvis
- failure to respond to a patient's call for help resulted in the patient getting up on her own and falling
- failure to appropriately train staff in transfer techniques resulted in a head injury when patient was being transferred out of bed
- failure to respond to a patient's request for help to get off a commode

Failure to use equipment in a responsible manner
- failure to use bed alarms and sensors
- failure to ensure that batteries were working in sensors
- failure to properly maintain a Hoyer lift, resulted in a fall
- failure to use a low bed
- failure to put up a side rail before rolling a patient on her side led to a fall off the bed
- failure to lock the wheels of a bed or wheelchair
- failure to ensure that doors to the outside or stairwells were not left propped open on units with cognitively impaired patient

Failure to communicate
- failure of the nurse to fill out forms instructing the aides on how to follow fall precautions for a woman with a previous history of a fractured hip
- failure to report a fall
- failure to instruct caregivers on proper transfer techniques

Failure to document
- failure to establish and record a plan to prevent falls in a patient with 57 falls and 18 head injuries
- failure to report and record details of a fall
- failure to record telephone orders for fall prevention measures

Failure to assess and monitor
- failure to monitor a patient who fell repeatedly ultimately resulted in loss of an eye during a fall in a parking lot
- failure to assess and monitor a patient following a head injury led to undetected increases in intracranial pressure and death

Failure to act as a patient advocate
- failure to report signs of lethargy consistent with over-sedation was followed by a fall
- failure to question excessive doses of psychotropic medications [16]

Critical thinking point for clinicians and legal nurse consultants: Cognitively impaired individuals represent the highest risk group for falls and are least likely to respond to corrective instructions from nursing staff. Many medical records will be replete with nursing notes reminding individuals to use the call button instead of attempting to exit the bed independently. When this instruction has failed for a protracted period of time without a change in the care plan, negligence becomes apparent. That is, when a specific mode of fall prevention strategy repeatedly fails, nurses are obligated to take proper steps to ensure that a new care plan is devised. [17]

E. Evolution of the Suit
The following steps typically occur following receipt of medical records by a plaintiff attorney.

1. The attorney scans the records, looking at the injuries the plaintiff claimed occurred as a result of the fall. The attorney reads the chart for evidence that the standard of care was followed. Some attorneys ask their legal nurse consultants to perform this task, or send the chart directly to an expert witness for review. A case usually needs two experts - a person who will assert that liability exists (someone did something wrong) and a causation expert. The physician is usually the causation expert, who will determine if the fall caused the injuries, and in a death case, led to the decline and death of the patient.

Critical thinking point for the clinician or legal nurse consultant: How do you know that an "assisted-to-the ground type of fall" did not result in any physical injury? What sources of data must be included in your comprehensive review to make this determination? Consider witness reports, review of x-ray or bone scan reports, and whether the injuries are consistent with the explanation provided.

---

2. The plaintiff's expert witness reviews the chart and advises the attorney as to whether a basis for a meritorious claim exists. The expert signs an affidavit of merit in those states that require it, and the attorney files the lawsuit in the form of a complaint. In some case, attorneys file the complaint before the expert has rendered an opinion. This is often done when there is a shortage of time before the statute of limitations expires.

3. The defense attorney and risk manager meet with the people involved in the incident and ask a series of questions. Refer to Figure 6-1.

4. The plaintiff's expert witness typically prepares a report (in those states that require them) and sends it to the plaintiff attorney. In particularly egregious cases, the case may settle before any additional discovery or work on the file has been completed. The plaintiff attorney sends the report to the defense attorney.
5. Attorneys exchange documents called interrogatories, which ask some basic questions about the case, and request documents, such as policies and procedures, incident reports, and so on. Expert witness reports are exchanged.

6. The defense expert is retained to review the material generated up to that point in the suit, including the report of the plaintiff's expert. This may include depositions of the plaintiff and nurses or physicians involved in the incident. The deposition is a fact gathering questioning that occurs under oath in the presence of attorneys for both sides and the court reporter. A transcript is made which is sent to the experts for both sides. The defense expert prepares a report if the case is defensible.

7. Expert witnesses may be deposed. Settlement negotiations may begin at this point. A defensible case is scheduled for trial.

8. Trial occurs anytime from 3 to 5 years after the suit is filed. A verdict may be appealed if there are grounds to do so, such as procedural error or errors made by the judge.

F. Defense Theories
The defense attorney runs through a checklist of potential defenses early in every case. These include the ones listed below.

1. Factual denial
To develop this defense, a meticulous review of the patient's prior medical records, facility chart, and physician records should be completed. A legal nurse consultant is the ideal person to perform this service. Additionally, expert testimony is needed to develop this defense. Some of the ways to deny the facts are listed below.

- The plaintiff attorney was mistaken when identifying specific nurses. The nurse's name was read incorrectly off the chart; or the nurse's name read correctly from the chart but another nurse gave the care; or plaintiff did not identify the nurse from a written record - the plaintiff attorney was mistaken.

Written notes contradict plaintiff's allegations. For example, the plaintiff claims the patient was in the bathroom at the time of the fall, but the nursing notes state the patient was found at the side of the bed.

Figure 6-2 Possible Fall-Related Questions Asked of Nurse Defendants by their Defense Attorneys.
Modified from Greene, P. "The Defense Attorney's perspective", in Iyer, P., Levin, B., Ashton, K., and Powell, V. (Editors) *Nursing Malpractice, Fourth Edition*, Lawyers and Judges Publishing Company, available from www.patiyer.com

Fall-out-of-bed cases: Questions asked of nurses
Do you remember this patient?
Was the patient on "fall precautions?"
Were you told in report about this patient?
(If the fall was out of bed):
Were the side rails up?

> How many side rails were up?
> What was the hospital's policy on side rails?
> Were bed alarms available on this unit and were they used?
> What was the patient's condition?
> Could the patient use the call bell?
> Did the patient have out-of-bed privileges?
> Did you observe the patient trying to get out of bed before the fall?
> Had you read the chart before the fall occurred?
> Did you review and update the plan of care?
> Where was the last time you saw the patient before the fall?
> How did you find out the fall occurred?
> Was there any history of confusion, restlessness or other risk factors?
> Was the patient on medication which altered consciousness?
> What was done on earlier and later shifts?
> What was your patient load?
> Where were you at the time of the fall?
> Were there any emergencies on your shift?
> How often did you make rounds?
> Did you fill out an incident report?

- An independent witness may contradict the plaintiff's story. For example, a woman asserted that she called for help and no one came to her hospital room. Her roommate testified that the patient did not call for help, and tripped over a telephone wire.
- The plaintiff's case relies solely on the plaintiff's own testimony and the plaintiff is not a reliable witness. For example, a case may involve an unwitnessed fall by a patient with some dementia.
- Plaintiff's case relies on the mere event without any corroborating testimony. For example, plaintiff was found on the floor and is unable to testify due to severe dementia.

2. Patient care or injury was the responsibility of others

- The physician was present at the time of the incident and made the medical decisions involved.
- The senior nurse was present at the time of the incident and made the nursing decisions involved
- The nurse did not have responsibility for the patient; other nurses who had responsibility were aware of the patient's condition at the time.
- The plaintiff injured himself in a different facility and came into the defendant facility with an undiagnosed fracture.

3. Recognized complications

The patient's injury could have occurred even in the absence of any negligence by the nurse, since it was a known risk of the patient's condition or the procedure being administered. This defense usually requires expert testimony and support in the literature. This theory might be applied if a pathological fracture occurred in a patient with metastatic bone cancer, for example.

4. Standard of care was followed

The most commonly used defense is, "We did everything right." This position asserts that the mere existence of an injury does not mean that the staff was negligent. Medicine is not an exact science and negative outcomes can result even when appropriate care is given. There are an immeasurable number of intangibles that can affect how a patient responds to the treatment or care rendered. Therefore, establishing that the facility met the standard of care required under the circumstances is seminal to this defense.

5. Nursing judgment

The nurse has some latitude in his or her actions depending on the facts of the case. Many situations are "a judgment call" and a healthcare professional should be permitted to exercise that judgment. For example, a nurse may assert that the patient acknowledged she understood the need to call for help when trying to get off the toilet. In the nurse's judgment, it was safe to leave the patient alone for a few minutes. Refer to Case Four in the Appendix.

6. Two schools of thought

Although an expert might testify that the nurse could have handled the situation one way, there is valid medical support for the nurse handling the situation another way. This requires expert testimony and, preferably, medical literature.

7. Lack of proximate cause

Volumes could be written about this defense. It is one of the most difficult concepts in law. The attorney argues that even if the nurse was negligent, the outcome would have been the same even without the nurse's negligence. As in any tort litigation, the plaintiff's burden is to establish that a deviation from the standard of care was the proximate cause of the injuries stated in the complaint. Since most older adult patients present with a multitude of illnesses and symptoms, it is often difficult to determine which of these have been preexisting and which of them may have caused a fall. [18] The notion of a fall as a prelude to subsequent illness has been cited in previous clinical research. [19] [20] In most states, establishing the proximate cause requires the testimony of a licensed healthcare professional. Depending upon the laws of the state in which the litigation occurs, the lawyer may need to utilize the services of a licensed physician since some states still do not recognize nurses as expert witnesses. Attorneys use both a nurse and physician expert in those jurisdictions that will not accept sole expert testimony from a nurse.

Examples of disputing proximate cause are listed below.

- The nurse was negligent in charting, but no one relied on the charting error so it had no effect on patient care.
- The nurse was negligent but the patient would have died of an unrelated condition anyway.
- The nurse was negligent but the negligence did not materially increase the patient's injury.
- The nurse was negligent but the patient suffered no harm as a result. The patient's hip fractured before he fell to the floor.

Typically the history and physical examination (when thorough enough to include a complete fall history, review of medications and pre-existing conditions) of the person who fell can aid the clinician in deciphering among potential underlying fall etiology. [21]

---

8. Contributory negligence of plaintiff

For the cases involving individuals who are cognitively intact, liability is typically quite difficult for the plaintiff attorney to establish. All regulations involving both hospitals and nursing homes place a focus on the responsibility of an institution and its nursing staff to ensure the maximum level of independence possible for an individual. In a practical sense, these regulations place fall related safety issues second on the list. These cases are appropriately defended on the basis that institutions, through their nursing staff, are compelled to ensure that otherwise frail individuals with significant comorbidities are nonetheless left free to engage in as many activities of daily living as their condition permits. This means that many types of fall prevention strategies, such as restraints, are not authorized. The significant exception involves cognitively intact individuals who are not capable of independent movement or transfers. A common presentation in this regard is the drop case when a patient is being transferred from bed to wheelchair, bath tub to wheelchair or wheelchair to bed. When it can be demonstrated that this individual was fully dependent upon staff for all modes of transfer, the nursing staff will have a difficult time or an impossible time defending the matter.

A competent patient has the right to refuse care. The medical record should contain detailed documentation concerning efforts to convince the patient to accept appropriate care. Competent family members with the responsibility of legal guardians may also refuse care on behalf of the patient. The concept of contributory negligence permits the defense to shift part or the entirety of the burden of responsibility onto the plaintiff. For example, if the patient fell while trying to get to the bathroom, the nursing notes may state that he or she failed to use the call light and wait for help.

The defense of contributory negligence can be effective in limited circumstances, such as:

- A patient failing to call a nurse when the patient was mentally competent and a call bell was easily within reach.
- A patient tampering with medical equipment, such as turning off a chair alarm or bed alarm
- A cognitively intact patient who gets out of bed or a chair or off a toilet without calling for help.

Severe limits exist on this defense, as follows:

- If a patient is under medical care due to a certain condition and a nurse fails to prevent a known risk to the patient from that condition, the nurse cannot invoke contributory negligence of the patient. For example, if a suicidal patient jumps out a window at the hospital, the nurse cannot blame the patient, when it was her duty to prevent this known risk. Likewise, if a feeble elderly patient is allowed to walk unattended and falls and hurts himself, the nurse cannot blame that on the patient either.
- If a nurse fails to perform a task or collect data as required, the nurse cannot claim that the patient is unable to prove he had the condition which the data might have shown if the nurse had collected it.
- Even without legal prohibition on the defense of contributory negligence, it is often a risky maneuver to blame an injured or ill patient for his or her own problems. Juries tend to disfavor this tactic.

9. Failure of plaintiff's expert to list a deviation from nursing practice

The failure of the plaintiff's expert to provide a comprehensive list of deviations is one of the key points of any defense. With few exceptions, such as the common knowledge doctrine or *res ipsa loquitur* (the thing speaks for itself). The only way that a plaintiff can prove negligence by a nurse is through expert testimony. If the plaintiff's expert, either in a written report, or affirmation, deposition testimony or trial testimony fails to articulate a particular deviation by the nurse, that deviation cannot be considered by a jury.

If a deviation is not listed as one of the plaintiff's nursing expert's opinions, the defense attorney should not elicit it at a deposition or at trial. The expert should be pinned down at deposition with the open-ended question, "Have you now set forth all the deviations from nursing practice that you find in this case?" Once the expert agrees that he or she has, the scope of trial is set. It is difficult for the plaintiff to add a deviation at trial which was not articulated by the expert previously. That is why it is such an important job of the defense counsel to limit plaintiff's expert opinions before trial. Any attempt by plaintiff to expand on his or her theories at trial will be met with strenuous objection, which will probably be sustained by the trial judge.

The defense team is also constrained to follow the opinions of their own nursing expert. The attorney will not be allowed to argue to a jury defenses which are not supported by expert testimony. That is why it is so important for the attorney to find a good expert and fully prepare that witness before trial. [22]

G. Punitive Damages

Punitive damages are those damages which are awarded to "punish" a defendant for substandard care beyond ordinary negligence. They are not covered by insurance policies and can be astronomical. Punitive damages are uncommonly granted in nursing malpractice cases. The lure of punitive damages from the plaintiff's perspective and the fear of said damages from the defense are a major part of any nursing malpractice litigation. Punitive damages must be pled in the complaint and must be explored early in the discovery phase of the lawsuit. There are three elements that must be established before a finder of fact is likely to award punitive damages: a continuing pattern of substandard care, a motivation for said continuing pattern, and substantial profits.

1. Pattern of substandard care

The continuing pattern of substandard care can be demonstrated in a variety of ways. First, the pattern can be established by evaluation of the individual plaintiff's case. For example, in a restraint-related death case plaintiff's attorney was able to produce medical records demonstrating a continuing pattern of substandard care. The nursing staff documented that the plaintiff attempted or successfully got out of bed either by removing her vest restraint or with it still attached to her at least ten times within a six day period. Unfortunately, the nursing staff continued to restrain her and the plaintiff did not survive her eleventh attempt to remove the vest. She was found unresponsive with a vest wrapped around her neck. This continued course of conduct by the nursing home was held by a jury to be beyond ordinary negligence and a substantial award (four million dollars) of punitive damages was rendered (*Case of the Estate of Minnie Viola Wilson vs. HealthSouth Corporation D/B/A HealthSouth Rehabilitation Hospital, District Court, Tarrant County, Texas, 96th Judicial District, Cause # 096-160043-95, 8/5/96*). [23]

The continuing pattern of substandard care as a basis for punitive damages may also be demonstrated with evidence of other patients who received substandard care. For example, there were an unusually high number of falls in a particular facility over a period of time that could be traced to a reduction in evening staff in order to avoid paying a shift differential. Another basis for punitive damages is to produce evidence that inappropriate treatment was given to a large number of patients. [24] For example, there may be a pattern of delayed medical treatment for patients who have suffered falls. Annual facility surveys required by Medicare and Medicaid and conducted by the state's certification or licensure agency are an important source of information. In addition to certifying facilities for Medicaid/Medicare, surveyors cite "deficiencies" which indicate non-compliance with one or more regulatory standards and issue violations and penalties based on the severity of the deficiency. The results of these surveys can be obtained from the facility or the state agency. It is apparent that establishing a continuing pattern of substandard care requires counsel to be diligent and sensitive to this issue during the discovery process. Any objections to this discovery should be quite easily overcome by arguing that they may lead to admissible evidence of a continuing pattern of substandard care.

2. Motivation to provide substandard care

The second requirement for punitive damages is motivation. In some instances the primary motive for substandard care is profits. However, there may be other motives. It is assumed that there are no motives of individualized malice towards any individual plaintiff. Any individualized malice would then become an intentional tort. This concept is beyond the scope of this discussion. However, there may be racial or gender-based bias which could also support a punitive damage award.

> It is unlikely that a trier of fact will be willing to render a punitive damage award if the defendant has not profited financially by the provision of substandard care.

3. Profits

The final requirement is profits. Accordingly, information relating to the profitability of the facility is essential. Usually discovery objections are simple to overcome. A plaintiff's inquiry, however, may not only be confined to the particular institution in which the plaintiff received care. Most healthcare facilities are affiliated or owned by larger companies. Accordingly, financial data may be obtained regarding the profitability of the entire company. The more a facility or chain has been shown to have profited from rendering substandard care the more likely a trier of fact will award substantial punitive damages. Moreover, the plaintiff attorney may seek to show that the profits from substandard care made this company or facility more profitable than either the industry average or other healthcare facilities that are not engaging in this pattern of care. Although the latter is difficult to prove, it will certainly increase the likelihood of significant punitive damages.

4. Defense of punitive damages claims

Conversely, the defense's objective is to show that if there was negligence, it was an isolated incident and not part of a widespread pattern of conduct designed to increase the facility's profits. While quality care given to other patients is generally irrelevant to. the litigated case, the skillful defense attorney may be able to maneuver plaintiff counsel into allowing the introduction of this type of evidence.

If there is an argument of individualized malice, the defense should take the position that this malice was unknown and is actively opposed. Evidence of thorough employee background checks and supervision of employees is persuasive in this area.

Conclusion

Falls occur across a spectrum of ages and within public and patient settings. The current body of evidence of fall and injury prevention research spans many age groups and settings. It directs us to interventions to reduce the burden of mortality and morbidity too often encountered from falls. The *Falls Handbook* provides you with the *tools* for ensuring safe practice and safe practice environments exist so that lives can be saved. Injury prevention, freedom from danger and reducing risk terminology are all synonymous with safety and the fundamental mission of quality healthcare. To sum it up, a quote by Robert Frost is reworded a bit and framed as a critical thinking point for you to consider, as you take this valuable knowledge we have presented in the *Falls Handbook* and implement it into your practice environment:

"How many miles are there to go, before you (we) sleep?"

End notes

[1] Cohen, D. "Screening the Nursing Malpractice Case", in Iyer, P. and Levin, B. (Editors) *Nursing Malpractice, Fouth Edition,* Lawyers and Judges Publishing Company, Tucson, 2011.

[2] Id

[3] Porto, G. "Disclosure of medical error: Facts and fallacies", *Journal of Healthcare Risk Management,* pgs. 67-76, Fall 2001.

[4] See note 1.

[5] The statute of limitations is calculated based on when the person knew or should have known that an injury occurred.

6 See note 1.

7 Id

8 Stevenson, D. G., & Studdert D. M. "The rise of nursing home litigation: Findings from a national survey of attorneys", *Health Affairs,* 22 (2), pgs. 219-229, 2003.

9 Holzer, J. F. "The advent of clinical standards for professional liability", *Quality Review Bulletin*, pgs. 71-79, 1990.

10 Cohen, E.S., and Kruschwitz, A.L. "Restraint reduction: Lessons from the asylum", *Ethics, Law, and Aging*, 3, pgs. 25-43, 1997.

11 American Geriatrics Society. (2002). *AGS position statement: restraint use*. Retrieved March 22, 2004, from http://www.americangeriatrics.org/products/positionpapers/restraintsupdate.shtml

12 Stolze, H., Klebe, S., Zechlin, C., Baecker, C., Friege, L., & Deuschl, G. "Falls in frequent neurological diseases—prevalence, risk factors and etiology", *Journal of Neurology,* 251(1), pgs. 79-84, 2004.

13 Mukai, S., & Lipsitz, L. A. "Orthostatic hypotension", *Clinics in Geriatric Medicine,* 18(2), pgs. 253-268, 2002.

14 Parker, K., & Miles, S. H. "Deaths caused by bedrails", *Journal of the American Geriatrics Society,* 45, pgs. 797-802, 1997.

15 Croke, E. "Nurses, Negligence, and Malpractice", *American Journal of Nursing*, 103 (9), pgs. 54-63, September, 2003.

16 Some of these allegations were extracted from review of nursing home fall cases published in *Medical Malpractice Verdicts, Settlements, and Experts* in 2001-2003 and were reported in Iyer, P., "Nursing Home Liability", in Iyer, P. (Editor) *Nursing Home Litigation: Investigation and Case Preparation*, Second Edition, Lawyers and Judges Publishing Company, Tucson, 2006, available at www.legalnursebusiness.com.

17 See note 1.

18 Miceli, D.G., Waxman, H., Cavalieri, T.C. & Lage, S. "Prodromal falls among older nursing home residents", *Applied Nursing Research* 7, pgs. 18-27, 2001.

19 Id.

20 Rubenstein, LZ., Robbins, AS. & Josephson, KR. "The value of assessing falls in an elderly population: A randomized clinical trial", *Annals of Internal Medicine* 113:4, pgs. 308-316, 1990.

21 Leipzig, R. M., Cumming, R. G., & Tinetti, M. E. (1999). "Drugs and falls in older people: A systematic review and meta-analysis II: Cardiac and analgesic drugs", *Journal of the American Geriatrics Society,* 47(1), pgs. 40-50, 1999.

22 Material in this section of defense theories comes from three sources: Cohen, D., "Screening the Nursing Malpractice Case", in Iyer, P. and Levin, B. (Editors), *Nursing Malpractice, Third Edition,* Lawyers and Judges Publishing Company, 2007, Greene, P., "The Defense Attorney's Perspective", in Iyer, P. and Levin, B., (Editors) *Nursing Malpractice, Third Edition,* Lawyers and Judges Publishing Company, 2007, and Myers, S. "The Defense Attorney's Perspective", in Iyer, P. (Editor) *Nursing Home Litigation, Investigation and Case Preparation, Fourth Edition,* Lawyers and Judges Publishing Company, 2006, available from www.legalnursebusiness.com.

23 Case of the *Estate of Minnie Viola Wilson vs. HealthSouth Corporation D/B/A HealthSouth Rehabilitation Hospital*, District Court, Tarrant County, Texas, 96th Judicial District, Cause # 096-160043-95, 8/5/96).

24 Marks, D.T. "Neglect in nursing homes", *Trial* 32, pgs. 60-62, 1996.

APPENDIX

Appendix One

Check for Safety: A Home Fall Prevention Checklist for Older Adults
Centers for Disease Control

FALLS AT HOME

Each year, thousands of older Americans fall at home. Many of them are seriously injured, and some are disabled. In 2002, more than 12,800 people over age 65 died and 1.6 million were treated in emergency departments because of falls.

Falls are often due to hazards that are easy to overlook but easy to fix. This checklist will help you find and fix those hazards in your home.

The checklist asks about hazards found in each room of your home. For each hazard, the checklist tells you how to fix the problem. At the end of the checklist, you'll find other tips for preventing falls.

FLOORS: Look at the floor in each room.

Q: When you walk through a room, do you have to walk around furniture?
Ask someone to move the furniture so your path is clear.

Q: Do you have throw rugs on the floor?
Remove the rugs or use double-sided tape or a non-slip backing so the rugs won't slip.

Q: Are there papers, books, towels, shoes, magazines, boxes, blankets, or other objects on the floor?
Pick up things that are on the floor. Always keep objects off the floor.

Q: Do you have to walk over or around wires or cords (like lamp, telephone, or extension cords)?
Coil or tape cords and wires next to the wall so you can't trip over them. If needed, have an electrician put in another outlet.

STAIRS AND STEPS: Look at the stairs you use both inside and outside your home.

Q: Are there papers, shoes, books, or other objects on the stairs?
Pick up things on the stairs. Always keep objects off stairs.

Q: Are some steps broken or uneven?
Fix loose or uneven steps.

Q: Are you missing a light over the stairway?
Have an electrician put in an overhead light at the top and bottom of the stairs.

Q: Do you have only one light switch for your stairs (only at the top or at the bottom of the stairs)?
Have an electrician put in a light switch at the top and bottom of the stairs. You can get light switches that glow.

Q: Has the stairway light bulb burned out?
Have a friend or family member change the light bulb.

Q: Is the carpet on the steps loose or torn?
Make sure the carpet is firmly attached to every step, or remove the carpet and attach non-slip rubber treads to the stairs.

Q: Are the handrails loose or broken? Is there a handrail on only one side of the stairs?
Fix loose handrails or put in new ones. Make sure handrails are on both sides of the stairs and are as long as the stairs.

KITCHEN: Look at your kitchen and eating area.

Q: Are the things you use often on high shelves?
Move items in your cabinets. Keep things you use often on the lower shelves (about waist level).

Q: Is your step stool unsteady?
If you must use a step stool, get one with a bar to hold on to. Never use a chair as a step stool.

BATHROOMS: Look at all your bathrooms.

Q: Is the tub or shower floor slippery?
Put a non-slip rubber mat or self-stick strips on the floor of the tub or shower.

Q: Do you need some support when you get in and out of the tub or up from the toilet?
Have a carpenter put grab bars inside the tub and next to the toilet.

BEDROOMS: Look at all your bedrooms.

Q: Is the light near the bed hard to reach?
Place a lamp close to the bed where it's easy to reach.

Q: Is the path from your bed to the bathroom dark?
Put in a night-light so you can see where you're walking. Some night-lights go on by themselves after dark.

Other Things You Can Do to Prevent Falls

Exercise regularly. Exercise makes you stronger and improves your balance and coordination.

Have your doctor or pharmacist look at all the medicines you take, even over-the-counter medicines. Some medicines can make you sleepy or dizzy.

Have your vision checked at least once a year by an eye doctor. Poor vision can increase your risk of falling.

Get up slowly after you sit or lie down.

Wear shoes both inside and outside the house. Avoid going barefoot or wearing slippers.

Improve the lighting in your home. Put in brighter light bulbs. Florescent bulbs are bright and cost less to use.

It's safest to have uniform lighting in a room. Add lighting to dark areas. Hang lightweight curtains or shades to reduce glare.

Paint a contrasting color on the top edge of all steps so you can see the stairs better. For example, use a light color paint on dark wood.

Other Safety Tips

Keep emergency numbers in large print near each phone.

Put a phone near the floor in case you fall and can't get up.

Think about wearing an alarm device that will bring help in case you fall and can't get up.

Appendix Two: Cases

The cases in this section are real. Comments are provided by Deanna Gray Miceli.

Case One: Inaccurate Description of Fall

An incident report was prepared explaining how a fall occurred in a nursing home. The incident report is shown below.

ACCIDENT/INCIDENT REPORT

Form #AS 1

REPORT OF ___✓___ ACCIDENT - An unanticipated occurrence, resulting in injury or hospitalization.
_____ INCIDENT - An unanticipated occurrence, resulting in superficial or no injury.

FALL: ☑ Yes ☐ No

Name: [redacted]   Room # 514A   Chart # 4083 B

Age 90   Sex F   Date of report 11·29·2000   Time 2:30 {☑}A.M. { }P.M.

Environmental Hazards, i.e., Wet Floor, Broken Equipment, Missing Shoes: Floor was dry and clutter free and Bed was Low Bed and Mats were on Floor

Location of Occurrence: Resident's Room 514A

Current Diagnosis: Fell from bed, sustained swelling on Lt. side of head & small skin tear on Lt. forearm. (CHF, A fel ert [illegible] CAD)

Mental Status: Alert ____ Forgetful ____ Confused ✓

Psychotropic medication: Yes ☐ No ☑ Specify Celexa 20 mg po OD.
Cardiotonic/Diuretic medication: Yes ☐ No ☑ Specify Digoxin 0.125 mg po OD
Restraint: Yes ☐ No ☑ Specify _____
History of falls in the past 3 months: Yes ☐ No ☑
Balance - problem while standing: Yes ☑ No ☐
Balance - problem while walking: Yes ☑ No ☐
[de]creased muscular coordination: Yes ☑ No ☐

The autopsy report cast doubt on the validity of the fall occurring the way it was described.

OFFICE OF CHIEF MEDICAL EXAMINER
CITY OF NEW YORK

REPORT OF AUTOPSY

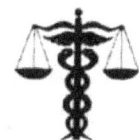

Name of Decedent: ███ M.E. Case #: ███

Autopsy Performed by: ███ Date of Autopsy: Dec. 1, 2000

CAUSE OF DEATH: BLUNT IMPACT INJURIES OF HEAD AND NECK WITH SUBDURAL AND SUBARACHNOID HEMORRHAGES, CEREBRAL SHIFT AND FRACTURE OF CERVICAL SPINE

THIS IS A TRUE COPY
Office of the Chief Medical Examiner
This record cannot be released without prior consent from the Office of Chief Medical Examiner, New York City, N.Y.

MANNER OF DEATH: ACCIDENT. (FELL FROM BED).

Comments on case
The veracity of the injury was questioned as there were two very different types of injury described - one on the incident report and the other from the description of the impact injury listed from the autopsy. The coroner described blunt impact injuries of head and neck with subdural and subarchnoid hemorrhages, while the incident report described swelling of the left side of the head and a skin tear to the left forearm.

Let us assume that this was a bed fall. The time of occurrence - 2:30 AM- is consistent with when a bed fall is likely to occur. However, the nature of the impact injury is not consistent with the interventions noted on the incident report. According to the incident report, the bed was in the low-position and mats were on floor. Floor mats used for the purposes of cushioning the floor surface from a bed fall are typically several inches of thick foam material providing an area of absorption (see Figure A-1). It was not mentioned if side rails were in place or not. If they were, the rails created a higher distance to the floor from a bed fall.

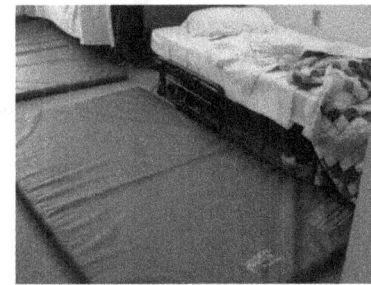

Figure A-1 Floor Mat

Critical thinking question for the legal nurse consultant: What injuries would you expect to find had the patient climbed out of or rolled over out of bed to the floor? Would you expect to find upper extremity injuries such as soft tissue damage or fractures to the shoulder, arm or wrist? Would you expect to find injuries lateralized to one side of the head or neck?

Thanks to Dr. Jeffrey Levine MD of New York City for the materials in this case study.

Case Two: Dropped by Aides

The woman was being cared for in a nursing home. Review the nursing notes below, which were transcribed verbatim.

2/6 8 AM	ABT continues in progress for TX of UTI. Received resident in bed awake and alert. Side rails up X4 and call bell in reach. AM care given. Pt transferred from bed to WC with assist x 2. Resident brings self to dayroom for breakfast. AM insulin given as ordered. Pt C/O pain in left foot. Medicated with Tylenol 650 mg per doctor order. Appetite excellent. Consumed 100% of breakfast. Fluids encouraged and tolerated well. Pt in dayroom for morning activities.
12 PM	No more C/O of left foot pain. Pt incontinent of bowel and bladder. Kept clean and dry. No C/L pain or discomfort upon urination. Pt brought self to dayroom for lunch. Appetite 100%.
2 PM	Patient put back to bed for afternoon nap. Kept clean and dry.
(no time)	T 97.2 ABT/UTI. Fluids offered. Taken fair. Voiding freely. Kept clean and dry.
2/7 2 AM	Resident C/O pain in right leg, hip and ankle when care is being done. Slight edema noted on top of right foot. Screaming when attempt is made to move right lower extremity. Supervisor made aware of resident's complaint and visited. External rotation noted of entire lower right extremity. Tylenol given for pain. Urine very concentrated. Fluids encouraged. ABT in progress for UTI.
5 AM	Still C/O some pain but not as bad as earlier. Temp 99.6 80-20
2/7 8 AM	AM care done by staff and C/O pain on the right leg when moved. Examination reveals no swelling and no bruise noted. Slight external rotation noted and C/O pain when trying to move or lift up right leg. Pedal pulses palpable.
8:30 AM	Called Dr. ___'s office and message left. 9 AM. Breakfast served in bed with HOB up and ate it well. Remained in bed at this time. 10 AM. Visited by daughter and daughter made aware of her C/O. She gets Tylenol tabs 2 (325 mg each) with offers slight relief.
11:30 AM.	Dr. ___ called in and orders received for X-ray of right hip, right upper leg, right lower leg, right foot stat! ABT cont for UTI, T 98.8. Flds offered, well taken as given. Inc. care done, turned and repositioned well in bed. SR up x 2 for safety. Consent signed by daughter. Care planning done and attended by daughter. Will continue present problem.
1 PM	X-ray ordered taken.
3 PM	Remains in bed, log rolling during change.
(no time)	BP 148/60, 97, 80 and 20. In bed awake and alert. Patient C/O pain in right leg. External rotation noted to right hip. X-ray results read Rt hip and Rt upper leg intertrochanteric neck fracture, right lower leg and foot negative. MD aware, family aware.

Comments on the case

The notes do not contain any description of a fall or incident relating to the fractured hip. Through investigation, the nursing supervisor learned that two certified nursing assistants were involved in dropping the patient while transferring her from bed to wheelchair. They did not report the fall and when confronted about the patient's injury, minimized the seriousness of what occurred. They described the injury as resulting from the patient's foot getting caught in the pedal of the wheelchair. The incident report and the statements of the aides follow.

[Incident report form, handwritten, dated 2/7/96]

Description of Incident: Resident reported to the undersigned that she had a fall yesterday in the morning when she was transferred from her bed to her wheelchair when I assessed her of her c/o pain on her upper thighs. Examination reveals no swelling, no bruise marks but noted slight external rotation of R leg and c/o pain when trying to lift up R leg from bed – unable to assess ROM to this leg due to c/o pain. Pt. is quoted as saying "I had a fall yesterday morning Mary and she left me in the room to get somebody to help her lift me up from the floor. I know they didn't tell you Mary!"

Initial Assessment: T 98, P 76, R 20, BP 124/72, Pupil Response PERL, L.O.C. alert, conscious, Grasp: good, R.O.M. good on both upper extrem., good L leg; unable to determine ROM due to c/o pain when lifted R leg, Pain: yes, R leg, Swelling: none apparent, Deformity: R external rotation (slight), Color: good

Nature of Injury: pain when R leg is moved

Follow Up Care / First Aid Admin: Use of leg rolling during care
X-Ray: Type R hip upper leg, Date 2/7/96

On 2/6/96 ▓▓▓▓ came to the nurses station in her wheel chair for her morning medication (like she does every morning) After giving her medication she told me that she had pain in her (R) foot so I gave her Tylenol per physician order. When I saw Y▓▓ W▓▓, CNA I asked her if ▓▓ had hurt her foot when she was being transferred from bed to w/c. I was told that ▓▓'s foot had slipped of the foot pedal while she was sitting in the chair. After she had been given the Tylenol she no longer c/o pain. On 2/7/96 during morning report we were told that ▓▓ was still c/o (R) leg pain & that her leg was slightly rotated outward. When T. W▓▓ CNA & V. D▓▓ CNA was questioned about ▓▓ they both had denied that ▓▓ had fallen. As of 3pm 2/7/96 neither V. D▓▓ & T. W▓▓ had come to me to tell me that Ms. T▓▓ had been injured during transferring from her bed to w/c.

M. ▓▓▓▓ LPN

INVESTIGATION OF INCIDENT FORM

NAME OF RESIDENT: [redacted] AGE: ___ TIME/SHIFT: 7-3 DATE: 2/7/96 RM. NO.: 314A

DIAGNOSIS: ___

REPORTED BY: Resident TO WHOM: M. R[redacted] RN

TYPE OF INCIDENT: BRUISE   ABRASION   (FALL)   OTHER
                   SKIN TEAR   ABUSE-VERBAL/PHYSICAL

EXHIBIT [stamp] P-280 ID 4/8/98

DESCRIBE WHAT HAPPENED OR WHAT CAUSED THIS INVESTIGATION TO OCCUR:
(WHO, WHERE, WHAT, WHY, HOW) Resident claimed that she had a fall yesterday morning when the aide was transferring her f. bed to w/c. She c/o pain in the upper thighs th affected her whole (R) L. Examination reveals no swelling nor bruise in her (R) thighs & hip but slight external rotation is noted in her (R) leg; c/o of pain when lifted up f. bed (R) leg) to assess hanging.

LIST DETAILS OF THE INVESTIGATION CONDUCTED: BE AS SPECIFIC AS POSSIBLE. INCLUDE ALL NAMES, DATES, TIME(S) OF INTERVIEWS AS NECESSARY. INCLUDE ALL STAFF INVOLVED. (USE BACK AS NECESSARY) I spoke c V. [redacted] CNA who had this resident as c/p 2/6/96 and she stated she didn't fall but she slide out f. her w/c but didn't report to the nurses. I spoke c T. W[redacted] who (over)

WAS THE RESIDENT ASSESSED FOR BEING AT RISK FOR FALLS (CHECK PRE-RESTRAINING ASSESSMENT) DONE (YES) NO

IS THE RESIDENT ON MEDS THAT MAY CAUSE INJURY? (YES) NO

WHAT MEDS: Serzone 100 mg. 1/2 tab. 50 mg. by mouth twice daily

TYPE OF INJURY AND ANY MEDICAL INTERVENTIONS NEEDED:

WAS THIS ADDRESSED IN C.P.? (YES) NO

WAS A NEW M.D.S. DONE? YES (NO)

IDENTIFY IF RESIDENT TRIGGERS RAPS FOR (FALL), (COGNITIVE LOSS/DEMENTIA), PHYSICAL RESTRAINTS, & PSYCHOTROPIC DRUG USE. (???)

DATE/TIME/NAME OF AGENCY NOTIFIED/PERSON REPORTED TO: 2/7/96 Dr. Y[redacted]   DATE/TIME/FAMILY NOTIFIED: 2/7/96

NAME OF EMPLOYEE ASSIGNED TO RESIDENT: V. D[redacted] CNA

STEPS TAKEN TO PREVENT FUTURE INCIDENTS:

COMPLETED BY: M[redacted], AN DATE: 2/7/96

REVIEWED BY: ___ UNIT DIRECTOR OF NURSING DATE: ___
[redacted] DIRECTOR OF NURSING DATE: 2-7-96
___ ADMINISTRATOR DATE: ___

---

is always her helping hand in a separate place & time c V. R[redacted] presence & she said the resident didn't have a fall but did slide down f. the w/c, not on the floor.

Comments on case

There are several important points to raise about this case They relate to failure of the professional nursing staff to assess the resident's complaint of left foot pain which originally occurred following a transfer from bed to the wheelchair on 2/6 at 8:00 AM.

Instead of properly assessing the foot pain in terms of onset, associated symptoms, radiation, ability to weight bear, the staff medicated the patient with an analgesic. This appears to be a cover-up given the fact that a previous body movement (transitioning from bed to wheelchair with assistance) took place. The analgesia worked in reducing the complaints of pain (as expected). Four hours later, there were still no reports of pain documented.

There was a failure of the professional nursing staff to assess the continued complaints of this patient's pain that progressed over 18 hours (from 8 AM on 2/6 through 2 AM on 2/7) and escalated. At 2 AM on 2/7 the physician should have been immediately notified of the new onset of swelling and extreme pain. Instead of doing this, the pain was placated with "Tylenol" and the supervisor, was notified. Still the supervisor failed to notify the primary care provider (an indication of a massive system failure). In the absence of an ability to make this telephone call, the supervisor and the nurse (2 individuals) did not even call for emergency transport to the hospital emergency department for someone else to make the assessment and order an x-ray. They failed to even relinquish the assessment to a competent provider. This delay could have had very serious health consequence for the patient, such as a fat emboli from fracture of a large extremity (which was later found to be the case) and death.

Transferring a resident requires special attention to proper body mechanics and knowing how to transfer without causing injury to either the patient or to the staff. There are many resources and aides to help facilities train staff and to ensure proper technique. This should be reflected in the policies and procedures as well in training logs.

Since the record indicates that although the patient was alert, she had disorientation and cognitive loss on a psychotropic medication, the staff might have assumed (incorrectly) that she was too confused to remember the incident or to follow through. This is an incident where the continued pain and ultimate swelling due to an extremity fracture speaks for itself (and can't be covered up). If the fall occurred in a corridor or public traveled hallway, hallway monitors, or video surveillance might deter this sort of negligent activity on the part of the staff.

Outcome: The case settled. The aides were fired.

Case Three: Fall Down Stairs

This is the case of an elderly woman who fell down steps in a nursing home. Her family requested that she be given a room on the ground floor because they were concerned that she would wander. Instead, she was placed on the second floor. These are the nurses notes transcribed verbatim.

Date	Entry
12/15 11AM	Admitted to W-9, family in attendance (daughter and husband.) Pt. alert, very forgetful, needs a lot of direction. Medication verified with MD. Eats in 2nd floor dining room. Appetite very good.
12/15 12:15 PM	Needs constant supervision or she goes downstairs or anywhere else she wants. Continuously walks unless told to sit down and rest.
12/15 7:30 PM	Nurse paged to West Wing first floor "stat" by first floor nurse. Found Mrs. _____ sitting on floor at foot of stairs, C/O of pain in right hip, right ankle and foot, rotated outward. MD called. Transfer to hospital for eval. Transported at 8 PM via ambulance. Adm and family notified.
12/21	Family notified adm that res will not be returning to facility after hospital stay. Family in to remove belongings.

Comments on case
The resident's family contacted an attorney after the fall. Questions raised include:

- Was the nurse negligent?
- What should the nurse have done once she observed the patient being in need of constant supervision?

Answers to questions with rationale:
In response to the question, "was the nurse negligent", the licensed professional nurse failed to follow an appropriate standard of care. The standard of practice for caring for an older adult in a nursing home requires recognition that wandering or getting lost can be related to an underlying organic problem of the brain, such as cognitive impairment due to dementia or delirium. This renders the person unsafe to make some sort of decisions that require judgment. Given that the patient was newly admitted and was wandering within the first hour of admission, coupled with the family reports of "getting lost" suggest that this patient was more likely than not experiencing some sort of cognitive impairment resulting in (short-term) memory loss. This observation is validated and consistent with the family members' reports of the resident has being forgetfulness and needing "lots of direction".

Although the patient was reported by the nurse to be alert, she was most likely none the less disoriented or confused (where the level of alertness remains intact). Level of alertness is distinctly different from cognitive impairment. If measures of cognitive impairment are included as part of the initial nursing assessment, such as a Mini-Mental State Examination, additional supporting data and evidence could corroborate the suspicion of cognitive impairment. In short, the registered nurse failed to recognize the importance of providing constant supervision to the patient given the reports by the family members and failed to utilize nursing knowledge that older adults admitted to nursing home are more likely than not suffering from memory disorders.

Additional records would need to be reviewed to determine if the nurse completed a comprehensive nursing assessment that included a cognitive assessment during the resident's evaluation. Remember that in licensed nursing home facilities, the nursing staff have up to 14 days to perform a comprehensive assessment. Having stated that, the admitting nurse is still responsible to ensure the safety of any newly admitted patient at the time of admission through the stay.

In response to the question "What should the nurse have done once she observed the patient being in need of constant supervision?" there are several possible interventions. These include (in no particular order of importance) one-on-one supervision through use of volunteer staff or assignment of a nurses' aide to stay with the patient. If facilities have in place wander-guard or other surveillance methods to prevent newly admitted residents from leaving the facility or a unit, these should be immediately instituted. It is imperative for maintenance of independence, function and mobility, that older adults such as this resident be allowed to move freely and ambulate on the unit *provided* she is supervised given the history of forgetfulness. A room change to be closer to the nurses' station is another option, particularly if there are more personnel at the nurses' station on a regular basis so the patient can be observed. But if the alternative room does not provide any additional supervision over the 24 hour period of time, then one should further question if this as a viable intervention.

All nursing and non-nursing personnel should be aware of the possibility that any older adult residents may become forgetful. Some facilities institute a colored vest or a special apron that residents wear indicating their potential to wander. Frequent environmental and room rounds that are documented on a checklist also help to identify residents who may be wandering off the unit. These are immediate solutions to the problem presented. But, consider situations where these types of incidences are occurring over and over again in the same facility. Lack of knowledge is not a defense against negligence.

Looking beyond the immediate circumstances of this case, consider if facility-wide measures of safety and fall prevention are in place. Certain immediate facility-wide responses and interventions are warranted after the fall incident occurred down the stairs to prevent another resident from doing the same thing. A closer inspection of the exit area and its condition is needed by members of the maintenance department coupled with risk management. Until a proper assessment is performed and corrective action taken, this area should be inaccessible to others. Important question include: are the steps and stairs structurally sound? Are there hand rails? Is there adequate lighting?

Outcome: The suit settled early on before any depositions were taken.

Case Four: Fall in Bathroom

This elderly female patient was recuperating in the hospital after a fractured hip. She fell in the bathroom of her room, fracturing her arm. After discharge, she sought a plaintiff attorney, who filed a suit against the nurses. The patient testified at her deposition that she went into the bathroom in the hospital room. When she realized she did not have toilet paper, she asked the nurse to get her paper. She testified that the nurse tossed the toilet paper at her, saying, "Here, catch!" She fell when she was trying to catch the toilet paper roll.

How do the nurses state the injury occurred? Refer to the verbatim nursing notes below.

Date	Note
11/30 7:30 AM	Awake and resting easily in bed. Suture line to left hip dry and intact. No drainage noted.
8:30 AM	Afebrile. VS stable. Breakfast taken fully. Intracath in right arm intact. No swelling noted. Voiding QS clear yellow urine.
10:45 AM	Dr. L____ vs. Dressing applied (dry) to left hip by Dr. L___
11:00 AM	OOB with walker and to BR for voiding. Pt states she was reaching for toilet paper and slipped and fell. Found patient on floor in BR lying on left side against tub. Left upper arm appears swollen. Dr. L___ present. NPO status now in effect.
12 PM	X-ray taken. Volpe cast applied to left arm by Dr. L____
1:30 PM	Re-x-ray done. Med for pain with Levo 2 mg SQ with relief.
3 PM	Brother vs. Hep lock now in right hand. Antibiotic infusing easily. Cast damp and open to air. Fingers cool and movable. Color good.
	Late charting
3:45 PM	Pt advised when OOB in BR to put call light on when wanting assistance. Assisted earlier to BT by ____ RN, also advised then to use call light when needing assist. When pt found on floor lying on left side, floor dry and uncluttered except for walker also lying on left side on floor. Pt seen in BR by Dr. L____ and then assisted to bed by G.___ RN and J___ LPN and Dr. L___
9:30 AM	Late note (written by a G___ RN, a different nurse) Assisted OOB for BRP. Ambulated well. Asked if she should put call light on. Told that she should put the light on for assistance
9:45 AM	Bathroom call light on. Stated "I was going to try to get up by myself but I know if I fell you girls would get in trouble." Reminded she was asked to put light on for assistance and should do so to avoid injury. Asst back to bed without difficulty.

Are the late entries written properly? (Yes, they were written the same day as the event, clearly labeled as late entries, and provide information which points to the negligence of the patient for not following instructions.)

Comments on case
What do you think about the validity of each side's version of the events? Do you believe the patient's version of events or the nurses' version? What additional information do you need to obtain and where in the medical record might you look for this information?

In attempting to retrospectively determine the validity of the patient's version of the story it is helpful to look to previous medical documentation about the patient's underlying mental status and level of consciousness at the time of the fall event. Was she observed to be alert, but confused or disoriented or was cognition intact and unimpaired? Were there previous statements in the medical record or a pattern indicating that the patient did not follow medical advice and chose to ambulate, get out of bed alone or unassisted against medical advice? Also consider use of medications affecting the memory and level of consciousness. Are there indications that the patient was taking medications that could cloud judgment or level of alertness?

This patient had a recent acute left hip fracture with surgical repair. She had the walker in the bathroom at the time of the fall. But what is unclear is her version of the fall event and where the fall occurred - on the toilet, near the toilet or outside the bathroom altogether. More information and clarity of existing information is needed, for instance was she sitting on the toilet or standing up before using the toilet when she realized there was no toilet tissue? If she was sitting on the toilet and made this discovery and called for help as she stated and was tossed a roll of toilet paper, she's likely to have fallen from a seated position to the ground floor. Injuries to the upper extremities would be expected such as those that did occur. But catching a roll of toilet paper tossed in the air from a seated position would result in one of two scenarios. Falling backwards while seated on the toilet would cause injuries to the spine and back of the head. Falling forward - lunging to catch the toilet paper- would likely involve impact injuries to the face, chin, neck or head as well as the arm. When the legal nurse consultant can either visualize or recreate the fall events step by step, additional information and possible scenarios can be explored as competing explanations for the injury. Note that hip fracture patients are typically prescribed an elevated toilet seat, raising the height of the fall distance to the ground surface.

Outcome: The plaintiff attorney dropped the suit, realizing that his client's version of events was not as credible as the testimony and notes of the nurses.

_____

Consider Writing a Review

Thank you for buying this book. When you enjoy a book, it is a natural desire to tell others about it. Amazon. com provides a way to share your thoughts and I invite you to write a book review. It is easy. Here are tips:

1. After going to the link below on Amazon.com, the first thing you are asked to do is to assign a number of stars to the book you think matches your opinion of the book.
2. Create a title for the review. This can be a simple phrase, like "Awesome guide." If you are not sure what to say, look at the titles of other book reviews.
3. It is easiest to write the book in a word processor and then paste it into Amazon.com Your word processor will pick up typos before your review goes public.
4. Write the review as if you were talking to another person – you are – a person who comes to Amazon.com and is considering buying this book.
5. Include a description of what you found most helpful. Was it an idea, chapter, tip? Share that with the readers.
6. Next you may want to write who you think would most benefit from this book. Is it for begin-ners? Or is it more appropriate for someone with experience with this topic?
7. What if you have something negative to say about the book? You may always reach me at patri-ciaiyer@gmail.com to suggest changes in the book.
8. If you include negative feedback in the review, keep a positive perspective rather than attack the author.

Here are some sample phrases:

- While overall the book was good, I would change it by. . .
- I don't think this book is right for. . .
- I would improve this book by. . .

Before you hit save, read everything over one more time.

Authors and readers appreciate book reviews and they get easier to write with time. Go to this link on Amazon.com to write your review. If for any reason it does not work, search for the book title + Iyer and it will show.

Link: http://bit.ly/FallsHandbook

Thank you,
Pat Iyer

www.ingramcontent.com/pod-product-compliance
Lightning Source LLC
Chambersburg PA
CBHW081238180526
45171CB00005B/461